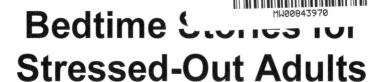

Bedtime Stories for Stressed-Out Adults

Fantasy stories and poems for stress relief and a good night of relaxed sleep. Lullabies for grown-ups.

Daisy Relaxing

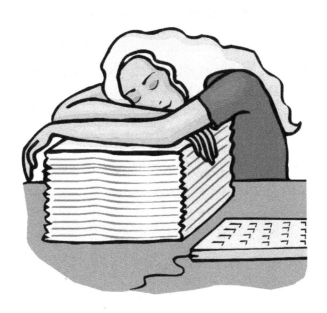

Table of Contents

By reading this document, the reader agrees that under no circumstances is the author responsible for any losses, direct or indirect, which are incurred as a result of the use of the information contained within this document, including, but not limited to, — errors, omissions, or inaccuracies.

Prologue

"Will you read me a story again tonight, Mama?"

"Yes, dear." Jenny lifted a large book and set it on her lap, its plastic slipcover crackling.

The book was old, as old as she was. *Adventures into Dreams* it was called.

It was the one her mother had read to her as a child, and once she had read as a young woman repeatedly. Each story transported her into another world, where dreams became reality, and the night became a place to meet all the things she had ever imagined.

She tousled the kid's hair and opened the book. Almost instantly, light spilled out, pale blue, white, and purple, and stars rolled along currents of wind and water. Kirsty's eyes lit up and she clapped her hands excitedly. Jenny smiled at her daughter.

"Tonight, I'll read you some of my very favorites. I went these adventures on growing up, through these stories, and the others. I think you're big enough now to really appreciate the magic of this book."

"Is it really magic, Mommy?

Jenny's eyes shone like a starry night sky.

"Yes, dear. Yes, it is."

She turned to the first page, which showed a stylized numeral "one" in the shape of a tree.

Around it was a forest of greens and yellows, and all sorts of animals hid within the painting.
Some of them looked up, listening to the distant forest sounds, before darting away into the undergrowth.

Some sat amid the branches and roots as the sunset painted the sky a brilliant maroon above.

"This story is about Jaina, the young woman who got lost and found herself at the same time."

"What does that mean, Mommy? Did she get scared?"

Jenny smiled. "Sometimes, she did. She is...she is like your mother, you know. But your mother when she was a young adult before she ever met Daddy or had you."
"So the girl in the story is you, Mommy?"

"Maybe, sweetie. Maybe she is you, too. I think whoever reads this book finds that the girl in the story, she's a lot like them, and when you're really in the story, it's a lot like having a good dream. It's hard to tell where one word ends and the others begin."

Kirsty laughed. "I don't get it, Mommy. I wish I got it!"

Jenny tucked the little girl in tight and smiled at her. "Don't worry, honey. You will. Now let me tell you a story...."

Chapter 1: The return of Jaina to the forest grove

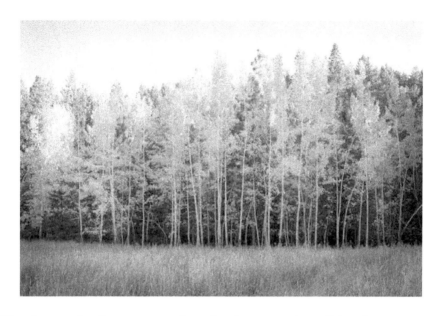

The forest shadows swayed as the Sun continued her lazy descent.

Jaina loved this time when things were starting to prepare for the oncoming night, but the buzz of late afternoon activity had not yet subsided. She walked barefoot in the grass, and along with the roots, and over fallen logs like mossy bridges across a stream.

Jaina had come here since she was a little girl, the advantage of having your backyard right next to the forest. Oh, of course, her parents had worried, but she was older now, she knew how to take care of herself. Besides, the forest was her friend. Her parents never understood that part.

A golden light shone down into the clearing. Green dust glittered in the rays that splayed through the leaves. Flowers bloomed in the clearing, blues, yellows, and reds in many hundreds, and an old stump stood in the middle of the clearing.

She did not know what had happened to the tree so long ago, but the old stump was not dead. Jaina had known that since she was a kid.

When she had first came here and sat on the stump, she could feel it living beneath her, telling her the stories of a long, long life in this place before ever there was a human voice questioning whether the trees really did make sounds when they fell!

As it turned out, the old stump had quite a lot to say quite a long time after he had fallen!

Colorful birds sang incessantly in the branches. Some of them stopped to look at her, to chirp a greeting, and Jaina waved. A light breeze tugged at her hair and her clothes.

She smiled and inhaled deeply. The air was so fresh in the clearing, in the forest. She stooped and smelled some of the flowers. Picking up a fallen red bloom, she set it in her hair and continued along the little glade until she came to the tree stump.

Sitting with her legs dangling over the edge (it had seemed so much higher up ten years ago), Jaina sat back on her hands and looked up.

One by one little pinpoint of white appeared in a deepening blue canvas above. A lone hare bounded into the clearing. It stopped and stood up, looking at her, and then it happily leaped away.

Then a fox appeared, going the opposite direction, but the fox stopped to talk to her.

"Good evening," said the fox.

"Good evening," said Jaina, and she smiled, and the fox smiled.

"Where would you be going tonight?" asked the fox.

"Oh, I don't know! I thought maybe I would just see what the forest was dreaming of tonight?"

The fox sat and lifted her nose, sniffing the air as if expecting something. "There is a lovely feeling in the wind tonight. I feel like sharing. Would you like to dream with me tonight?"

Jaina's eyes lit up. "Yes, I would! I've always wondered what foxes dreamed."

The fox laughed. "Then place your hand on my head and I will show you."

Jaina hopped down from the stump and approached the fox. She wondered if she should be afraid, given the fox's reputation as a trickster, but something in the air told her to simply run with it. A cool, comfortable night was coming and she wanted to dream as the fox dreamed.

She placed her hand on the fox's head, her fingers threading through warm fur, and the fox laughed. "Heed no nightly noises, for tonight we dream together!"

Then Jaina leaped away in the body of the fox, and the forest came to life.

A shimmering green light seemed to emanate from the trees themselves, pulsing softly as if in tune with the heartbeat of the land itself.

Jaina the Fox saw motes of glowing green: fireflies, they were, but bigger and brighter than any she had ever seen. Their light created a piece of music, and all things danced in tune with the music.

Flowers swayed on their stalks. The branches above waved back and forth and the leaves fluttered, turning colors like butterfly wings and then flying away.

The Fox felt the music of the forest so keenly. Perhaps that is why she was so amused: to her, every moment was like a waking dream, and now Jaina got to feel a part of that. She felt like a part of the forest itself, of the endless green and growing things.

Along the paths, she darted, swifter than the hares that fled her coming, nimbler than the squirrels that skittered up the trees. As she ran, she grew to know the forest as the Fox knew it: paws on the earth, wind in the fur, the taste of freedom upon her tongue.

Night veiled the forest in deepest blue. The lights danced in the trees and guided her way. There were dangers, to be sure, the night-spirits and the ancient ones that walked the deep forest, but they could not catch her.

She was the Fox, too quick and too sly for anyone to catch her. Because she knew the tune for them all, and it gave her a sense of guidance as she bounded through the woods. Fox had the quickest feet and the quickest wits. She had never been caught yet in many long, long years, and she was not going to be now.

Jaina felt that confidence and sense of utter peace. Union with the land itself, with the dream, with both waking and sleeping worlds, flesh and blood, root and sap, real and fantasy.

She was part of this great music, familiar on the most primal level, at once the most ancient and yet always a new scent, sound, taste, feel. She knew the sheer joy of darting from bush to bush, path to path, racing into a whole night of potential.

Howls went up into the night, as the wolves closed in, but the pack came not as enemies.

She ran among them for a time, fellow travelers in the forest night-dream. For that span, the only sounds were of panting breaths and paws thumping on the earth in time with the land's pulse. They were all one, a glimpse of the sheer exultant joy of life in its most primal incarnation. Blood thundered. Voices howled.

The night was alive around them. Spirits capered in the wind and half-hidden in the shadowy eaves. Some looked on with laughter at the passing four-legs, some looked on with envy, but none could match their sense of pure freedom.

The moment passed and the Fox went her own way, accompanied by howls of kinship from the wolves. For she had far to go yet before the Sun rose and dispelled the magic of the night.

The deep forest was a place of the most ancient and primal dreams. Here stood trees that had outlasted ages of the world, groves that had long ago disappeared in the waking world but remained hale and bountiful here.

They were sustained by and embodied the very dreams of the land itself, a time of rampant growth and viridian tenacity. When they sang, their voices were deep and hollow, ringing far out over the land, heard by every leaf and stem. Needles danced upon the forest floor at the vibration of it, and leaves upon the branches fluttered happily.

Shadows were deep beneath the tall trees but they hid no malice nor dangers. The deepest heart of the forest was a place of pure growth, where the biggest of the trees would count its rings greater than the number of leaves in the forest.

Each of the mighty trees bore an entire world upon its branches. As a fruit, these visions hung a globe, storm, and an ocean in a single drop. If one dropped, it burst into being and filled all the dreams of the forest.

From root to treetop, the great trunks emanated this music of creation, bastions of a time when the world was young and its harmonies still coming together.

As the Fox, she bounded happily through these forest depths, privy as few sleepers were to the powerful sounds of the most ancient of living things. The land itself spoke through these guardians, and all who would know the truth of the dreaming earth could listen.

Few experiences were more transformative, and Jaina on her own may have lingered for a lifetime or several just to listen.

"It is truly amazing," said Fox. "You are fortunate. Not many can hear this music conducted from the heart of the forest. It has the power to shape the world itself."

"I know," said Jaina, her voice hazy as though caught in the spell of sleep. "It's...old, but ageless. Like a new pebble breaking off a mountain. Alternatively, a drop from the waterfall. It's part of something impossibly old, but also touches you like it was brand new."

Fox laughed. "You speak well, friend. This is the song that courses through the lifeblood of the world. What you feel when your feet touch the warm grass in the summertime, or you smell the air after a rain, or you feel the breeze that blows warm through the forest. This place is the very embodiment of that feeling. Life is at its strongest here, and its dreams are the most potent."

Jaina could have spent forever soaking up that potency, but she had so much more she wanted to see.

Together with Fox, they hurtled roots and fallen branches and leaped across shallow ravines. They passed clearings where the sunlight never left, even at the deepest of night.

Those were places where the world had been awake for so long that wakefulness and dreaming were the same things. Tinged with the primal essence of living history, the sunlit clearings warmed Fox's fur but she hurried through them.

"There are other places I want to show you yet before we see the Sun again!"

The paths that led through the forest would have left most travelers hopelessly lost, wandering in the great emerald beauty of the forest until they awakened.

The Fox was sly and she knew the paths better than anything did that ran on two or four feet. She could not so easily be lost, even in the depths of the forest. Over hills and across ravines upon moss-covered fallen logs she darted, swift and sure.

Her nose lifted into the air sometimes to snuff out the path, or her ears flicked as she stopped to listen, but she always found her way. She had run the forest for many long years, and she would continue to do so for many more to come.

At last, the canopy thinned again and she came to less wild parts of the woods. She came to a stream bubbling and gushing along a well-worn path. The Fox turned her course, running alongside it for many miles.

The stream spoke to her as it rushed and burbled along its path, envious of her ability to choose her own path, carrying hundreds of voices from distant lands.

"Hello!" said the Fox to the stream. "Are you cold and swift tonight?"

"I am cold and swift," said Stream, "but I carry many dreams! Maybe one will warm you?" The temptation was there, to jump into the icy water and be carried along as part of its endless stream of dreams and voices.

"Not tonight!" laughed Fox and she jumped clear over the stream. Its voice faded behind her as she ran into the deeper forest and raced up a great grassy hill.

The top of the hill reached just above the treeline so that it seemed to be a green head crowned in trees. All around her Fox saw a sea of deep green, faintly illumined by silver starlight above, and green earthlight beneath.

"This! This is the greatest view in the forest. But this happens only in the deepest hours, just before the Sun returns."

Then Jaina was herself again, beside the Fox, and looking out upon the same amazing view. There was a single broad stump on the top of the hill and she sat upon it, dangling her legs, breathlessly admiring the incredible vista. Like every dream, the forest had ever had woven into one perfect tapestry.

"So, do you regret running with me?" asked Fox.

Nevertheless, she already knew the answer that never came, because Jaina was fast asleep, curled up on the tree stump, and sleeping more soundly than she had in many years.

Fox smiled, for she had long to go yet, but Jaina's part of the journey stopped here for now. She had many more to undergo, more dreams to find, but tonight, Jaina slept as the forest itself did.

Fox darted into the shadow of the woods.

Fireflies danced in the air above Jaina, who dreamed of running like a fox through the magical night-forest.

* * *

"Did you really get to sleep in the forest with the foxes and the trees and the fireflies, Mommy?"

Jenny smiled. "Yes, dear. Now, tonight you will get to do the same thing." Nevertheless, the little girl was already asleep with a slight smile on her face. Jenny tucked the blankets in around her and shut off the lights, pausing to look at the fireflies and the fox that lifted her head and smiled at the foot of Kirsty's bed.

The Gloaming

Tis the time between the hurried day, and the peaceful night.
The burdens are put away and slumber is in sight.
Time to settle with a book and a cup of tea
Moreover, let your mind drift and wander free.

As the day, from night slowly divides;
Enter the 'tween time where Magic resides.
Take a deep breath, and gently relax
On the wind, the subtle scent of roses and lilacs

Walk with your mind in the garden of dreams
Where nothing is quite as it seems
With a fluttering eye and a nodding head
'Tis time to slip off to the comforts of the bed.

Time to dance until the coming of the morn
With the whimsical dreams that were born
In the magical Gloaming; the sweet twilight,
Rest peacefully into the sacred midnight.

Dreamscapes

Nightly, through the dreamscapes, I travel
Letting the stresses of the day unravel.
I walk the hidden paths of my imagination
My mind in deep contemplation.

Be it a dune on a forgotten beach,
Recalling a memory just out of reach
Or a tranquil forest at twilight
Catching glimpses of wildlife just out of sight

My mind wanders among the world of dreams
Running in meadows and wading in streams
I dive unfettered in an underwater cave
Then rush up to meet the crashing wave.

Lighthearted as a child, I chase fireflies
Magic beings of light, they mesmerize
I watch for a while, and then gingerly I set them free
Gracefully they float away, up and over, beyond the Rowan
tree.

Nightly I wander a dreaming vagabond
Exploring the mystic worlds beyond.
Returning each morning, I awake

To the majestic beauty of a new daybreak

Moonrise

I sit and watch the moonrise
Awaiting her appearance in the inky skies
Behind the mountain begins to show
At first just the faintest glow

Then appears the tiniest sliver
The anticipation makes me quiver
Ever so slowly, she ascends
To the night, her grace she lends

She leaves the mountain below
Her full glory now does show
She travels through the night
Bathing me in her magical light

Earth Walking

Treading upon the earth with bare feet
The feel of moist dirt between my toes
Here is where I feel complete
Mother Earth, she soothes all my woes.

Treading upon the earth, I find the soul
When I feel depleted, she helps me rejuvenate.
It here where I feel whole
And all my problems abate

Now Comes the Springtime

Now comes the Springtime, like the opening of a blooming
flower
The sun grows warmer with each passing hour
The birds, emerging from their slumber, being to sing
And the wind chimes, in the breezes begin to ring

The grass spouts green and new from the earth
And baby animals emerge soon after their birth
Flowers slowly open and peak out to face the sun
Closing again, to sleep when the day is done

Now comes the springtime when everything begins growing
And all of the rivers, are swollen and flowing
The warmth and light are once again returning
And for this, my soul has been yearning

Waterfalls

Down to the waterfall, I go to refresh my soul
To cleanse my heart and make my spirit whole
The water refreshes and cleanses
So, I can see the world with new lenses

The rush of the water brings much delight
And the falling stream makes prisms of the sunlight
Cool water rushing from the mountains above
Bringing my inner being laughter, light, and love

Dancing in the roaring water, as it showers
Here I shall be for hours and hours
The waterfall is my secret, happy place
Sitting here I forget everything else in time and space

Midnight Stroll

She went on a midnight stroll
Through the forest to the hidden knoll
Where the fairies were rumored to play
And there she watched for the Fae

She was not disappointed, as one by one
The wee folk came out of the mound for a bit of fun
They giggled and the danced upon the grass
She determined only to watch till the hour did pass

But the Fae are a tricky race
Time for them is nothing, humans cannot keep pace
Before she knew what to do or say
She woke up realizing she had been watching for a year and a
day

Chapter 2: The ocean

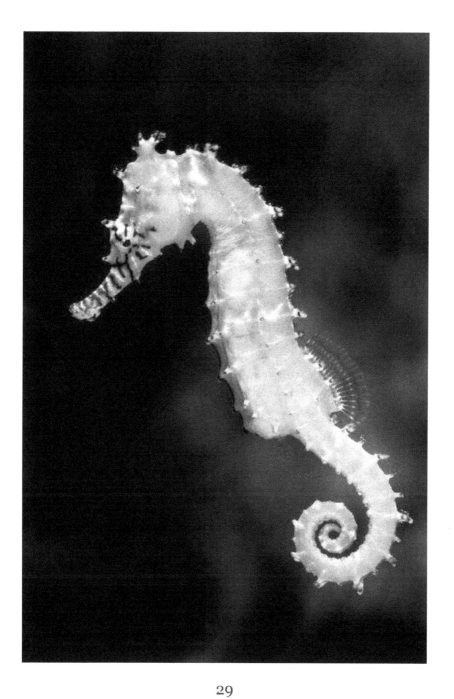

Kirsty clapped her hands excitedly. "Tonight's another one, right, Mom?"

She held the large book in her little hands, positively shaking with enthusiasm as Jenny sat on the bed. "Which one is it tonight?"

Jenny took the book and opened it to another chapter. The painting showed a stylized numeral "2" in the shape of a seahorse.

Behind it was a colorful coral reef standing over a seabed: reds and oranges and blues and greens, bright fish swimming among swaying seaweeds, an eel winding its way in and out of the reef, a crab crawling across the silt.

As they looked, bubbled streamed out of some hidden opening in the reef, and the crab darted to safety as the eel came looking for it. A school of fish obscured the view before disappearing in a rush of bubbles.

"Yes, baby, this is one of my favorites, too. Did I ever tell you about that time I got to swim with the dolphins?"

"You did? You really did?"

"I did! But this is your story now." Jenny smiled and tapped the picture, which showed in the background a pod of dolphins playfully darting through the water. "See? I think that one kinda looks like you...."

* * *

Jaina walked along the beach. The sound of gulls crying in the air overhead greeted her, mingled with the sibilant lap of the waves upon the shore. White sand stretched before her in a seemingly endless squiggle. No one but the seagulls to keep her company.

She breathed in deeply, smelling the salt in the air, closing her eyes, remembering how she used to run barefoot upon the beach as a child. The sand still felt just as warm and comforting to her toes now as it did then. She knelt and brushed her fingertips through the sand, picked some up and let it slide through her fingers.

The sun shone brightly upon the gleaming waves. Jaina approached the water's edge, foaming as it lazily crawled ashore and then slipped back again.

She remembered that when she was a kid, she had a friend here, one of the many dolphins that sometimes swam near the beach. They jumped, flipped, and spun merrily and she always wanted to be out there with them.

Once, she swore, the dolphins let her swim with them, but of course, her parents had never believed her. No one had, but Jaina knew the dolphins were her friends. They let her be one of them for a little while.

Now that she had moved back home, Jaina wanted to swim with the dolphins again, but they seemed to be gone. She had come to the beach hoping to see them, but she was mostly alone this morning.

Well, Jaina could make the most of it. She laid down in the sand on her back and waved her arms and legs to make a sand angel...or a fish, she thought, as she looked at it. No, now it looked more like a dolphin. Yes, that was it, a dolphin splashing happily amid the waves.

The imprint was so lifelike she could nearly hear the high-pitched cries of the dolphins.

Wait, it *was* them! Jaina turned happily out to the ocean and saw the silvery creatures flipping and rolling as they breached the waves and gleefully plunged back down again. She called and waved her hands. One of the dolphins seemed to notice her, and it swam closer to shore, gracefully diving from wave to wave.

"Hello, my friend!" cried Jaina, wading out into the water.

"Hello, my friend!" said the dolphin, lifting its head above the water. "How you've grown! I did not recognize you!"

"I could never forget you," Jaina said, beaming. "The star-marks on your fin and your voice are forever in my memory!"

"You have been gone for many years, but we are here still, and we swim from sunrise to moonset! Will you swim with us again?"

Jaina laughed joyously, and for a moment, she had forgotten about the intervening years. "Yes! I wish to, more than anything does! I want to remember what it was like to swim in your world!"

"Then come with me," said Dolphin, and he turned and dove into the waves. Jaina followed, and soon she found that she swam not as people do, but with fin, fluke, and perfect grace. She was swimming as Dolphin, and together they raced through the water with the sound of sloshing and thundering underwater pressure.

The other dolphins welcomed them back, knowing an old friend had rejoined them.

Jaina was now in a dream come true, she was Dolphin, and they swam together with Dolphin's people.

The pod raced away, soon leaving the shore behind and flying through the water far out to sea. Above them, the seabirds circled but they were in their domain, and *this* world belonged to Dolphin. This morning, it was Jaina's, as well.

Sunbeams shone like blades down from the surface. The dolphins frolicked amid the golden shafts of light, dancing together through the morning.

A warm wind tangy with salt whipped the surface of the waves. A school of brightly colored fish scattered as the dolphins approached.

Some chased them, their clicks and high-pitched cries signaling hunger and the thrill of the chase to the rest of the pod. Others let them go; they were too busy, they said, having fun chasing one another and tasting the morning in the water.

As the sun moved through the sky, the dolphins swam a little lower. They loved playing among the reefs not far from the shore, where the most magical colors were found.

Coral of burnt red and sunny orange nestled amid rocks and rolling hills of silt.

Some dolphins went down and kicked up clouds of silt with their tails, and then played hide and seek with each other among the clouds.

Still, others were curious about the many things that inhabited the reef.

Dolphin Jaina, for example, saw an old turtle swimming past. Floating up to the turtle, Dolphin chirped a greeting.

"Hello!" said Dolphin, "and where are you going this morning?"

The turtle was old and cagey, but not so, old he could not answer with one eye fixed on Dolphin. "Good morning! I am going home. It has been a long time now since I walked on the shores of my origin, and I want to see them again."

"The land?" said Dolphin. "What a dry place! Give me surf over sand any day!"

"I have known both," said Turtle, "and often when I have one, I long for the other. You are young and do not know the call of the other world yet, but give it time. You may wish you could walk as I do."

"And you may wish you could swim as I do! Good day!" With that, Dolphin sped away, leaving the old Turtle to shake his head and continue on his journey.

Dolphin rejoined the pod, whose chatter had grown quite excited in the frenzy of their play.

After all, a warm current wound its way through the reef and brought with it a sense of excitement and possibility. A deep, inviting blue surrounded them, a perfect canvas to be painted silver with the dolphins and many yellows, greens, reds, purples, all the colors of the reef.

Groups of bubbles erupted from the activity and floated toward the surface, and each one contained a dream-like Jaina's. For the dolphins were carriers and friends to many; the Ocean was a place of pure dream.

Those that slept on land came here in their dreams, and those who dreamed in the water embodied the eternal ebb and flow of life here.

"Let's go deeper!" Dolphin cried as the Sun sank a little in the sky.

Alternatively, perhaps it just grew darker the deeper they went. Out beyond the reef lay a strange and endless land where the ocean floor fell away in great canyons, and the plains of silt and seaweed stretched on forever.

There were big fish here, shining like their scales were made of diamonds. They did not flee the dolphins; nothing deterred them on their slow cruise for food, but they had little to say.

The dolphins soon gave up on trying to get them to play.

Big, bulbous jellyfish undulated through the water. Some of them glowed, shimmering light blue and red in hypnotizing waves. Several dolphins circled around them, admiring their translucent bodies and luminous patterns.

The jellyfish said little, a constant song, a hum, their voices ancient and speaking of older things the young dolphins did not understand.

Great beds of kelp floated and swayed in the currents. Eels and gleaming fish floated among the soft green stalks. Small sharks swam with single-minded determination, looking for their next meal.

The dolphins, as a rule, did not try to play with the sharks, because the sharks rarely had anything interesting to say. Instead, the dolphins capered around them, drawing their cold envy at the sheer freedom they enjoyed the day in and day out.

The kelp had its own voice, a long song of growth. The song began deep down in the very roots, speaking of the things that crawled in the slime and muck upon the ocean floor, and as it rose, many other things became entangled in the words: currents, fish and jellyfish, even the light itself.

The tall kelp had seen it all over the course of its long life and it knew the voices of so many things.

A shadow passed overhead as something blotted out the light filtering in from above.

Long, beautiful notes rang out.

Whales passing through, majestic giants who roamed from one blue horizon to another.

They shared in the sheer joy of the dolphins, exulting in the embrace of the mother ocean.

But their perspectives were far-reaching, slower, as they swam slowly through the world.

The dolphins called to them, and the whales called back.

Dolphin swam to one, a great blue, its eye shining with many years of experience.
Its body was like a reef unto itself, and around it, the very ocean streamed and rolled a royal raiment to fit an old queen.

"Greetings!" cried Dolphin. "You are so vast and beautiful; looking upon you is like looking upon the ocean itself!"

"Thank you!" answered Blue. "How I wish I could join your little ones as you frolic above the waves. But this is my home and I love her so. Tell me: have you heard our songs?"

"I have! We love them so. We wish we could dive as deep as you!"

"And I wish I could fly as high as you! You are very young. Depth will come to you yet. I may never fly, but as long as I can dream, I will dream of your people."

"Nay!"-said Dolphin. "For you are the very living dream of all things in the ocean. Your majesty is unrivaled."

Blue smiled, and the whale slowly swam on, her mountainous form vanishing into the gloom.

Dolphin laughed, following her for as long as he could, but soon he had to return to the pod—and Jaina with him.

A cacophony greeted them: the dolphins and their endless chatter, but also the swift hums of schools of fish, and the tiny, high-pitched voices of the little things that crawled along the ocean floor.

Before they stretched on a landscape where seaweeds, kelp, and little coral formations wove a tapestry amid the blue depths.

The dolphins were but one group in countless who all joined their music to that of the ocean.
Over the silty hills there lay a treasure: a sunken ship, its timbers coated in the muck, its mast still jutting tall, sails full of holes but still billowing in the current.

This was the dolphins' favorite playground. An old galleon, which had lain upon the bottom for ages and ages, but it, had become a part of the ocean floor now.

Little shelled creatures made their homes in the bowels of the sunken ship.

Fish circled its upper decks, finding a sense of calm in its long restful sleep.

One lone octopus floated near a yawning hole in the ship's hull, and Dolphin greeted it courteously.

"Many-armed friend! It is long since I have seen you!"

"Good afternoon!" sang the octopus, waving its many arms.

The two of them floated into the ship's interior, find it coziest next to a broken chest full of gleaming golden coins.

The octopus settled onto the bed of coins and laughed. "This place is still nice and warm. Would you like to stay here for a nap?"

"I can't," said Dolphin, "because we have a long way to go still to get to the islands. But I will peak in on you when we come back this way."

"Farewell!" The octopus settled onto its golden bed and soon grew still with peaceful slumber.

Past the sunken ship and its creaking timbers, the ocean grew wide, darkening slowly as the sun began to sink.

The dolphins swam back for the surface, admiring a deepening orange sky over gray-green waves. Water splashed and sprayed around them. The sound was soft and relaxing, the sleepless voice of a dreaming ocean. Far on the edge of sight, islands like mountains rose up out of the horizon.

"That is where we will go," said Dolphin. "There are many new dreams to await us there. But for tonight, we will sleep here."

Night rose up to stain the sky darkest blue, stars shining like pearls.

The dolphins dove beneath the surface of the water, where silvery rays pierced the veil.

All below them was a cloudy blue gloom, but they could still hear the music of the night-fish and the seaweeds.

Somewhere in the distance, the long and sonorous songs of the whales drifted to them, lulling the dolphins one by one into sleep.

"Are you glad you came back?" said Dolphin to Jaina, but she was fast asleep, on the beach, lying upon her blanket and dreaming of azure depths and ancient songs.

Dolphin smiled, and he turned to his people, swimming lazy circles around them until at last he, too, fell into a dream. And he dreamed of turtles walking upon the white shores, and of Jaina, with her hair streaming in the sea breeze.

* * *

Jenny ran her fingers through her daughter's hair. She turned off the light and stopped to look at the aquarium on the vanity near the bed.

A sunken ship held a small treasure chest, spilling golden coins onto the aquarium floor. A small octopus had taken up residence there, still as though it was made of ceramic....

But as Jenny turned to go, the octopus waved to her, and Jenny waved back.

Midnight Ocean

Moonlight glistens upon the ocean waves

Through the night, air dances a balmy breeze

Night birds are calling, hidden in swaying palm trees

Take a walk along the shoreline

Foaming waves rushing up to greet

Bringing soothing refreshment to tired bare feet

The ocean at midnight, alive yet solitary

A sanctuary for the anxious soul

A journey to becoming whole

Mermaids

Mermaids dive and play in the ocean deep

And the steal away to a hidden grotto to sleep

Days the spend playing and searching unfound treasure

Evenings they sit on a rock, singing for nature's pleasure

Swimming with a school of fish in a spiral dance

Then on to a darkened cave without a backward glance

With not a fear, they stealthily swim inside

Exploring in wonder the place where bioluminescent creatures

abide

Mermaids live in a magical, secret, hidden place

That no human eyes may ever grace

But should you be walking upon the shore at the day's end

Listen closely for you may hear their song on the wind

Lost in the Dreamworld

Lost in the world of dreams
Where nothing is, as it seems
Do take a road with no end?
Can all of my beliefs suspend?

This surreal world of nighttime visions
Is one without reason or precision
I walk, I fly, I swim, I float
I have been out to sea, minus a boat

A world with a different reality
But full of excitement and vitality
A realm created by the imagination
Creativity is its only explanation

Chapter 3: A tropical island

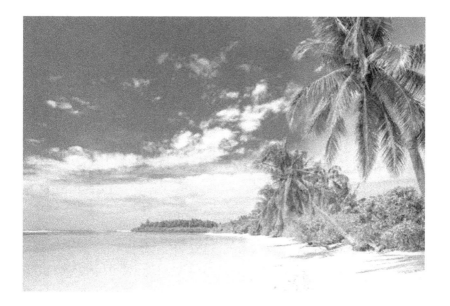

"Can ee fim wif da dolphins 'gain, Mommy?"

"Finish brushing your teeth first!" Jenny called into the bathroom.

The silly child poked her head out of the bathroom, toothbrush in hand, lips covered in toothpaste.

"Okie, Mom!" Flecks of toothpaste flew as she said it, and then grinned with foamy teeth.

Kirsty came out wiping her mouth with the back of her long sleeve and hopped into the bed as Jenny pulled back the covers.

"I really like the dolphins, Mom. They know how to have fun!"

"They do." Jenny nodded. "But there are all kinds of dreams to explore, you know. There is an entire world full of them out there. All kinds of perspectives you never imagined."

"What does 'perspective' mean, Mommy?"
Jenny tapped a finger to her lips. "It's...it's a way you view the world. Do you know how you got to see the forest dreaming from the fox's view? That's a new perspective."

"Oh, okay! So what kind of per-spec-tive are we going to see tonight?"

Jenny opened the book, it is cover crackling. She flipped through the pages until she came to the next chapter.

"Oh, yes. This is a special one."

She turned the book so that Kirsty could properly see the picture.

It depicted a tropical island, thick with palm trees and ferns, and fallen coconuts on the beach forming a pattern that looked like the numeral "3."

Above it, in the swaying branches and green canopy, peeked all sorts of brightly colored birds.

Their many calls mingled with the sound of the lapping waves to create a light and hopeful background.

The scent of salt and the pungent fragrance of tropical plants drifted from the pages.

"Now, sweetie, let me show you what the dolphins were so keen to get to explore, but from a different perspective...."

* * *

Jaina woke up on a beach, but not the beach she had left.

Now instead of a sandy path back to the city, she found herself on a tropical island.
Coconuts littered the sand at her feet.
Bright red and spiky fruits hung in some of the trees.

A warm tropical wind blew past, stirring the leaves with a whispering rustle and billowing her hair.

Jaina smiled as she breathed it in. The air smelled so fresh, a lingering tang on her tongue.

She turned toward the nearby jungle.

A small bird with green feathers and a shiny blue around its head hopped down from one of the branches. "Welcome!" it chirped. "This is my home. Do you like it?"

Jaina nodded enthusiastically. "It's wonderful. So warm and cozy and peaceful. How do you ever stay awake here? I think I would spend my day napping if I lived in such a nice place!"

"Oh, but you don't know what else there is to see!" said Bird. "You would have no time for napping all day if you could see the beauty of this place!"

"Could I? Could you show me?" Jaina looked hopeful, her eyes big and bright. A bird could not resist her plea.

"Yes, I will show you. Come with me and see what only one on the wing can see! Then you tell me if you would spend all day napping."

"Deal!"

Jaina held out her arm, and Bird alighted upon it, tilting its head back and forth to stare at her with each eye.

"And…let the wind takes us!"

Then it flew off again, and Jaina found that she was looking at the beach from high above.

She was like Bird, winging her way through warm blue skies to appreciate the jungle and the ocean from on high.

She circled higher and higher, and the whole island became a green-carpeted seed below her.

Up until this high in the sky, only the winds kept her company, singing of the distant waves, of the past and the future.

"Here we go!" Bird dove down, tucking her wings, as the green jungle rushed up to meet her. She spread her wings and arced smoothly into level flight, circling the treetops.

Below her, she saw the coconuts sitting in the trees, humming softly in the breeze.

Harsh voices rose up to meet her: monkeys leaping from branch to branch, picking the fruits and eating them with lyrical delight.

They looked up at Bird as she flew past and waved their hands in envy.

Into the canopy, she plunged.

Green fan-shaped leaves fluttered in the wind as she flew past.

Other birds, some of them yellow with black beaks, and some of the dark blue with yellow beaks, and still others red with white markings sang loudly, all competing voices.

They looked up as she flew past. Some rose into the air with a flutter of feathers, but they could not keep up with her speed.

She wove through corridors of green and tan, leaves and branches adorned with fruits or coconuts, nimbly winging around tree trunks, dodging hanging vines, and great big spiderwebs glistening with morning dew like living chandeliers.

The chorus of chirps and hooting cries followed her as she raced through a blur of the jungle.

Then she was free and flew out over the beach, above the water. Fish leaped and swam in the cerulean waves, all aglow from the sunshine warming the world.

Dolphins cavorted off the shore, leaping high from white-capped waves to glisten in the sun and crash back down again.

Bird Jaina watched the shadows darting about beneath the surface, and then she turned back to the island.

Flocks of seabirds circled on the shores, diving down to peck at some meal washed ashore.

"Food! Food! Food!" their cries said. The bird had more on her mind than simply eating.

She circled the island, white sand streaming by beneath her, the lush jungle rotating slowly in her eyes.

Slender fingers of sunlight crept through the canopy and golden dust swirled in their grasp.

Little lizards and dark beetles crawled up the trunks, racing to the top to reach the sunlight. Their voices rose ever higher in competition.

The bird let out a warbling song to drown them out. Her voice echoed in the jungle as she spiraled ever higher, eventually reaching high above the island once more.

"This is an amazing view!" said Jaina.

"Yes, it is." Bird tucked her wings and dove once more. "But sometimes you need to see from a bird's eye view up close!"

Down she flew into the jungle canopy, landing upon a high branch.
The wind caressed her feathers as she preened her wing, and then looked down on the world unfolding below her.

In the thick undergrowth, many creatures crawled, each with a voice of its own.

A furry anteater hummed its slow, ponderous song as it wandered lazily through the brush, long tongue flicking out of its long face. The anteater stopped and looked up at Bird as she sang down to it.

"Good...morning..." said the anteater, it is every word drawn out and rolling.

"It is a good morning!" said Bird. "But there are no ants up here, my friend."

"That's...okay." The anteater plodded along on its search.

A soft croak drew her attention, followed by another, and another.

Small frogs with very vibrant coloring hopped up the tree trunk.

Bird knew better than to test them: they were beautiful but dangerous if you were careless, much like the sweetest of dreams.

One of the frogs, neon green with red sides, leaped from the tree as a wind sighed through the palm fronds. The frog spread into wings of luminous glass, a butterfly with glowing blue and black patterns on its wings.

As Bird and Jaina watched the butterfly shattered into a hundred tiny slivers of blue light, and each grew wings, a sudden swarm of sky-blue butterflies shining in the shaded forest canopy.

Laughing, Bird flew down to join them, and suddenly found herself caught within a cloud of swirling blue. They spiraled with the wind, down nearly to the ground and then back up into the branches, pushing through the leaves and emerging into the sunlight beyond.

As the butterflies flew, a symphony of fluttering notes filled the air. The bird stopped flapping her wings and for a moment just drifted up on the music of the island itself: the rush of wings, wind, and waves, all joining together to create a warm sound.

The frond-leaves were as wings, emerald feathers joining her in flight. Whole flocks rose out of the green to take to the sky with her, and they soared so high even the wind envied them.

Blue skies opened up before them, and to Jaina's delight, she found they soared higher still. Into kingdoms of cloud they flew, where mountains of mist and moisture rolled past, and visions of the ancient world rose up and fell away in mere moments.

Clouds became like islands in the sky, floating upside down in an airy ocean.

The wind rolled through it all like oceanic currents, some warm and lazy, some cool and swift.

The flock changed again, leaves borne upon the wind, now clad in white cloud-feathers, wreathed in a scent of rain.
Thunder rolled and the islands gave way to a downpour, cascading from the clouds as waterfalls.

The flock dove into the rain, becoming like fish of sea green, fins like wings, but the music never changed. The song of the island: that of sea and sky, where the voices of the waves and the dreams of the wind combined.

Therefore, down they fell, back into the water, bursting through the surface and emerging from a geyser of bubbles in yet another world. There the deep blue embraced them, warm and salty, and they sank into its liquid softness. Currents enveloped them.

Colorful ocean fish darted back and forth amid the reefs that surrounded the island, and the flock changed yet again, becoming like them, bright and quick, yet trailing seaweed from their tails. Longer and longer, the trails grew, as they flew through the water around the island, binding it in green.

The land became green beneath them, and the clouds of fish were as clouds in the sky, glimpsed through the shimmering surface above them.

Green seaweed beds settled onto coral and melted together into trees with palm leaves and the rocks that once adorned the reef hung from the trees like coconuts.

Sun shone through the surface, upon which the shadows of swaying trees danced.

She landed beside a pool in the center of it all that slowly filled up with clear gleaming water.

The bird looked into the pool and Jaina was there beside her, staring at their reflections.

She sat back and laughed. "That was amazing!

I never knew the island was so perfectly poised between the two worlds."
"Three," said Bird cheerily.

"Earth, sea, and sky. This little island offers them all for those who want them. Even for one who has hopped and flown every single inch of this island. Do you see now why I never tire of it? To nap here would be divine, but if this whole place is like a dream come to life, would you need to?"

Jaina sat back on her hands. The warm tropical air stirred her hair and tasted faintly of salt. She smiled.

"I think it would be hard to tell the difference. This entire place is perfect. As you said, it's got something for everyone."

A coconut fell and rolled down a little sandy hill, bumping lightly into her knee.

Jaina picked it up and found that it already had a straw in it, drawn from the little reeds that surrounded the pool.

She sipped at the sweet coconut milk, the taste rolling over her tongue like the white clouds through which they had flown. Jaina lay back on a bed of soft, fragrant tropical flowers.

Closing her eyes and just relishing the tastes of the island, Jaina did not even notice the coconut slip from her fingers.

The birds continued their endless cries around her, and the wind continued to caress the waves.

Jaina fell into dreams that were little different from the waking beauty that was the island life.

Bioluminescence

In the waters of the darkened deep
A world of magical creatures swim and creep
Jellyfish undulating, glowing blue, purple, or green
Unnamed creatures never before are seen

Creatures of living light, so impossible to believe
A thought one would never conceive
Brilliant underwater light show,
A million, swimming fish all aglow

Glowing plants too, swaying with the ocean waves
Along the sea bottom and lighting up underwater caves
The magic of this place, as the sea creatures float and shimmer
A haven of peace for a weary soul; a dreamtime swimmer

Dreams and Sea Glass

Once, alone I went to the shore
Looking for sea glass but found something more
There were the land meets the sea
I was found by a kindred soul, and he spoke to me

He said "Hello" and we talked for a while
Of our dreams and places, we had been, and then we shared a
smile
One thing neither of us could possibly know
Was how in time this friendship would grow

Little by little their dreams our dreams we would share
And slowly, day by day we started to care
In time, he became a best friend none could surpass
Walking along the shore, sharing dreams and sea glass

Mirror

I wish I had a mirror to reflect
To show you yourself, in circumspect
That you could truly see the soul inside,
And look at yourself with pride

I want you to know, how beautiful you are
To see that you can do so much; go so far
To know the gentleness, you possess
And to see, that you can be a success

I wish I had that mirror to show
So you could see and you could know
That you are amazing, talented, and smart
That you have a poet's soul and a golden heart

The Wind

The wind kisses my cheeks and it blows by
It lingers for a moment, then leaves; no one knows why
The wind whispers its secrets to the trees
Then blows away in a playful breeze

Leaves dance, and whirlwinds blow
The wind, delighting us with her show
A whimsical elemental friend
Ever changing, ever-present. The Wind.

Chapter 4: Grandma's farm

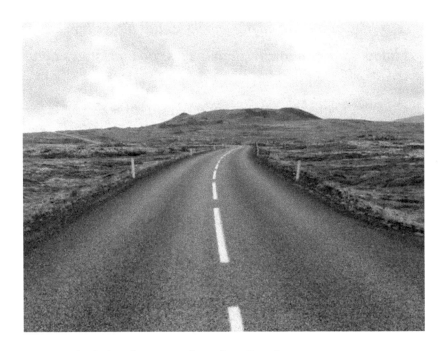

Jenny needed the drive to clear her head.

It had been a long week. Her boss was breathing down her neck and at home, Kirsty was competing for attention with a nine-month-old baby.

Her husband was also working long hours and often out of town, leaving Jenny to handle the kids, coordinate the bills, and do all the chores.

Sometimes she just felt like her neck was so tense she could barely turn her head.

Always another unexpected issue to pop up, always something going wrong.

That was life, she told herself, but it did not make it any easier when she was up all night fretting over a looming bill or an appointment.

These drives out in the summer afternoon were a wonderful way to clear her head. She would call her sister and have Aunt Julia come and watch the kids while she sometimes went out for a few hours just to think.
On the other hand, she would even bring Kirsty and the baby with her, out to the old country roads outside the city.

Sometimes she would even drive back as far as the farms where she used to go and visit her grandparents, even staying whole summers out there. Helping to till the fields, plant the crops, or feeding the animals (which was always her favorite). And the nights!

Listening to the steady voice of a distant creek, and the soft roar of wide-open spaces.

The occasional bleating of an animal or the long, mournful-sounding cries of the peacocks. A rush of feathers as a bird flew overhead, returning to its nest to sleep. The playful thumps of the barnyard cats coming indoors for a meal and to chase one another.

A wide expanse of grass and golden hills opened up before her, slowly drifting past.

The road dipped and rose again, winding its slow way out through the countryside.

Sprawling patches of tilled fields and growing wheat gave way to beautiful farmhouses and old, weathered barns in the distance.

She wondered what it would be like to live in such a place, enjoying the fresh air and the night skies full of stars.

Her grandparents had so often said it was the single best thing they had ever done, making the move out to the country.

While Jenny loved her life, its many challenges made her long for something simpler.
The afternoon grew warmer. White puffs of cloud lazily floated through a cerulean sky.
Jenny found her mind wandering back to some of her favorite days as she drove through a corridor of tall trees on either side.
A little excitement built in her belly, just like it did when she was a child, because on the right side of the road ahead, the treeline

thinned out and then stopped, and as soon as it did one could see her grandparents' farm down at the end of a very long gravel driveway.

Every time she drove down this way, her heart did a little leap as she approached that last tree lining the road.

There it was! A small white patch glimpsed in the distance, across wide fields, standing amid other buildings: an old barn, the ruins of an old house now used for the chickens (and the cats), a hay shack, pens for the pigs, cows, and horses.

She saw the cows in the field, though they looked like small black and white lumps from this distance.

It had been a few months since she had visited Grandma Belinda and she decided now was as good a time as any.

Grandpa Dale had passed a few years back but had his ashes mixed with the soil of the farm fields. He always wanted to be a part of the growth and lives of that place he loved so much, and even as she turned down the long driveway, she saw he felt his warm smile beaming upon her like the afternoon sun.

The gravel crackled beneath the car tires. Long before she would ever get close to the house, the dogs' ears would perk up and they would go running and barking home—or out to meet her once they recognized the car.

There they came now, barking excitedly as they rushed across the field to meet her, while she had to take the driveway around the long bend and finally past the older buildings to the farmhouse itself.

Jenny rolled down the window and smiled as the dogs kept pace with her car, barking their greeting.

"Hey there! Did you miss me, guys? Go and tell Grandma that I'm here!"

And as if they had understood, the dogs did turn and ran back for the house, but Belinda needed no warning. There she was standing in front of the house, now walking out to meet Jenny as she drove up.
Grandma had a layer of dirt and grime on her clothes; she had already been out that day working somewhere on the farm.

The woman was a marvel in her ability to keep going, even despite her age when Jenny felt like she could barely muster the energy to get through her own challenges.

"Grandma!" Jenny was quick to greet her grandmother with a hug.

Belinda smiled as she embraced her granddaughter.

"It's good to see you, dear. I have been thinking about you lately, you know. I was hoping you'd come to visit soon!"

Jenny then knelt and played with the dogs, one a rambunctious Border Collie, the other a mutt with the most joyous wagging tail any dog had ever known. They flopped and rolled on the lawn before her, so excited they could barely contain themselves long enough to be petted.

Jenny laughed, and as she did so, weeks of worry and stress that had built lines upon her features smoothed away, weight lifted from her shoulders, none of it ever to return.
The sheer joy of being out here, in the warmth and sun, while the entire mountain around them bloomed, overcame any hardships.

Deep shades of green filled all of her sights, as the mountain rose still further up in the distance, and a steep incline led down to a little creek valley behind the house.

The forest was at its height of growth in the fullness of its Summer. The smells of fresh water mingled with the scents of evergreen, the heady aroma of wheat, even the unpleasant animal pen smells were tied to memories.

The whole experience was a life unto itself, a story that unfolded anew each day with the crowing of the roosters to green the dawn.

A peacock sounded off in the tree above the old house that had been converted into a chicken coop. Several others also howled in response.

Jenny loved that sound now, but when she was a kid, she thought it sounded like they were saying, "Help! Help!" A light breeze stirred her hair and gently rumbled in her ears.

She took in a deep breath through her nose and let out a long and satisfied sigh.

"Grandma, it's so good to see you. I went for a drive and I just ended up here. I thought I'd see how you were doing."

Belinda smiled. "I was just about to go and give the animals their dinner. Do you want to help?"

"Do I?" Jenny's eye lit up.

Feeding the animals was always her favorite part as a kid. Grandma knew that. She nodded toward the animal pens. "Come on. I already knew the answer to the question."

The dogs followed the women as they walked around the farmhouse toward the pens.

Grandma asked Jenny about her life, and Jenny told her how things were going.
She tried to make it sound like everything was fine, but Grandma had keener ears and eyes than that.

"I know you're stressed, sweetheart, but trust me: you're doing well. You've got a great family and you're making it work."

"I just feel like it's so much of a struggle sometimes, you know, Grandma? Is it normal to feel this way? Like you don't have it under control?"

Belinda chuckled. "Yes, honey, it is. In fact, I would be more worried if you said you did not even have to worry. However, you are doing what you should be doing. Raising a family on your own isn't easy, but it's also the most beautiful challenge you'll ever experience."

She opened up the weather-beaten door of a large shack, and the smell of animal feed drifted into the air.

"You just have to remember that no one controls it all. It is okay that you cannot do anything. And it's okay to take some time away to get a new perspective."

Belinda handed Jenny a large metal cup, which Jenny gladly scooped into the animal feed. Dust swirled upward as she brought the now-heavy cup up full of feed pellets.

She followed her grandmother out to the pigpens and poured the feed into the troughs, and then back to the shack to do it again.

The horses and cows also received multiple cups of the feed, but then Jenny and her grandmother-retrieved armfuls of hay from the shack and tossed them over the fences for the bigger animals. Soon all were crunching happily at their food.

One of the horses, a big mottled silver and white horse named Bingo, came to the fence.

Jenny had named him in her creative youth, shrilly singing the song as she did so, of course, but he had always been a favorite of hers. She gently patted the horse's forehead and snout, and he thanked her with a thunderous snort.

Bingo went back to the food, while Jenny returned to her grandmother.

They walked along a trail past the house and down to the converted coop.

Rusted tractors derelict for many years sat in the tall grasses, and other things like mossy, decayed wooden fences added the weight of history to the trail.

The sun began to sink a little, disappearing over the forested mountain, casting its light but not beating down upon them. The air-cooled and carried with it a sense of freshness and vitality.

Jenny thought she could breathe in that air forever.

"You know, you're a lot stronger than you think, Jen."

Belinda looked over at her granddaughter as they walked.

"You realize that you've been smiling this whole time? Just like when you were a girl. Same lopsided grin and everything."

"Aw, Grandma."

"It's okay to feel overwhelmed or frustrated, dear. However, the important part is this. What you are doing right now. Taking some time to let it all go. To reconnect."

"I wish I could live out here all the time. I do love the city, but this is so much more relaxing."

Belinda looked around, her gaze sweeping across the entire plot of land.

"It *is* nice, dear, but its work, no matter how you look at it. That is what we do. We take care of our families until they don't need us anymore...."

But Grandma smirked as she turned back to Jenny, who grinned wide.

"But they *always* need us!"

"Exactly."

Their footsteps thumped on the floor of the old house as they walked in to feed the chickens.

A heat lamp shone over the nesting box where the chicks chirped. One wall in the front room held shelves of boxes for the hens to lay their eggs, and branch-like perches in front of them. Straw and feathers covered the floor.

Jenny loved the sounds the chickens made; the constant soft clucks and squawks had always been very relaxing to her.

The women spread the chicken feed on the ground just outside the door, and some in the hen room. Most of the chickens gathered around them and followed them outside, recognizing their feeding time.

Jenny crouched down and reached out slowly to pet some of the chickens that came close. They were docile and friendly creatures, and some of them looked at her before moving on to their food.

Jenny closed her eyes and listened to the sound: the scratching of their beaks on the ground, the soft flutter of their feathers, their clucks telling each other of the food they found. Peaceful. Simple.
Grandma's hand rested upon her shoulder.

"Even this, my dear Jen, should remind you. The chickens do what we do. Even now, they are calling to the others, telling their young of the food they have found. They are taking care of each other. Because that is a hen's job, dear. Our jobs are never finished! You just have to take that time to appreciate all the simple things, and *be* appreciated."

She held out a hand to help her granddaughter up.

"Come on. Let me make you dinner. It is our turn to eat. Then you can drive back and sleep a little more easily tonight."

Jenny took the proffered hand and they walked together back to the house.

Grandma cooked up a lovely dinner, and they shared stories, laughed over old memories, and Belinda gave her a parting gift.

"This horseshoe was the very first one I ever put on a horse. I did not know what I was doing. I was young like you, scared; worried I was not doing anything right. And you know what? All these years later, I kept this because of it as a reminder that I *did* get through it. That I was stronger than I thought. Now I want you to have it. And I want you to remind yourself every time you feel like you are not good enough that you are. You can get through it, too."

Jenny accepted the gift with tears in her eyes.

She thanked her grandmother many times.

The two of them shared a long and reluctant goodbye after dinner, and although Jenny hated to leave, as the sunlight receded from a clear sky and the fresh air rolled in through her window, she drove home with a lighter heart.

The road was empty but for Jenny and her dreams of a better life. Dreams that she was working every day to foster, just like the chickens, just like her grandmother did.

The night was pleasantly cool and welcoming as she drove, settling like a blanket upon the fields and the forests.

She checked on the girls. Julia had fallen asleep while reading Kirsty a bedtime story, and the baby was asleep in her crib. Jenny gently caressed the baby's cheek, then turned out the light and went to turn the lights out.

The house settled into the quiet hum of the peaceful summer nights. Jenny paused to listen and had the feeling that her grandmother even now was doing the same thing.

When she laid down in her bed that night, Jenny dreamed of chickens and peacocks, riding over the open fields beside a stream that softly murmured to her with her grandmother's reassurances. Summer night sounds drifted in through the window, along with the distant whinnying of a horse.

Fire Dancers

I see the dancers in the fire
In the flames, spiraling higher.
Spinning to their cracking song
Fire dancers, my mind dances along.

Fire dancers, burning all the night
Smoldering to slumber in the first morning light
For my forgotten frivolity, they make me yearn
Beautiful fire fae, will you return?

Frogs and Pollywogs

When I was a child, I found such delight
In frogs and pollywogs
When I would go down to the pond to play
I would forget my games and watch them all-day

How does this little swimmy, fishy thing
Become a creature that can jump and sing?
So much time I spent in contemplation
And my days I spent in anticipation

Now my days are filled with adult responsibility
That I have forgotten all about possibility
When and how it is not clear
But somehow the magic, it did disappear.

I think today I shall run away
And go back to the pond where I used to play
I sit on the wet, mossy logs
And spend the day watching frogs and pollywogs.

Summer at the Farm

I want to go back, for one more summer on the farm
And spend my afternoons on the front porch shelling peas
I will drink sweet tea and gossip with grandma and Aunt
Louise

I will go out and hoe weeds from the garden
And pick green tomatoes to fry in a cast iron pan
The tomatoes will be lined up on the counter ready to can

Grampa will be out in the field on his tractor
Cutting down, and then bailing up the hay
All to ensure his cows have food some snowy winter day

When the sun goes down, Grandma will ring the dinner bell
And later we will sit on the porch and watch the fireflies
And then we shall retire, only to wake with the sunrise

If only, I could have one more summer on the farm
But all I have now are the sweet golden memories
That comes to my thoughts as gently as a summer breeze

Chapter 5: Dandelion wish

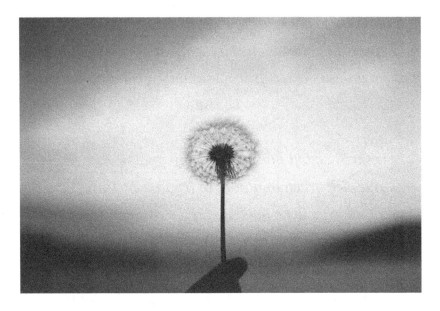

The summer was as gorgeous as any Jenny had known.

Days of running through the sprinklers, and going out to the lake, and having picnics in the local park.

Roasting marshmallows in the fire pit out in the backyard, making s' mores, and enjoying family get-togethers around the barbecue.

The weather was warm but cold lemonade and shade under the trees helped to keep everyone cool.

Jenny worked hard and brought about many changes: remodeling the home, taking on a new role at work, helping her daughter recover from her very first exciting school year.

Tonight, Jenny sat with Kirsty out by the fire pit in the fading evening light.

The others had gone inside, but she wanted to spend the night with her daughter and enjoy one of the last nights of summer.

The smell of wood smoke drifted on the air. Gentle pops and crackles accompanied the embers that floated up in the air, glimmered, and went out.

One of Jenny's favorite things in the whole world was to sit next to a fire and enjoy the warmth and flickering glow, and the sound, the smell, all of it. She loved it, and now she had passed that down to her daughter, as well.

The steady sound of crickets and the occasional hoot of a night bird made a relaxing chorus to lull their heavy eyelids ever down further.

"I want a story, Mom," said Kirsty, yawning heavily in her chair. Then she hugged the blanket she had brought outside even closer around her.

Her head leaned back, but she was not ready yet. Jenny had brought out a sleeping bag because sometimes they liked to sleep out under the stars, on perfect nights like tonight.

Kirsty got out of her chair, went over to the sleeping bag, and slid into it, the fabric swishing loudly as she snuggled in.

Jenny moved her chair over near the sleeping bag.

"I thought you might, honey, so I came prepared!"

Jenny lifted the book she had had sitting beside the chair: their favorite storybook.

"How are you going to read in the dark, Mommy?"

The flickering firelight did not offer much steady light for reading, but Jenny only smiled.

"Oh, don't worry, baby."

She opened the book and turned to one of the summer chapters, and a golden light spilled out from the very pages, illuminating Jenny is smiling face.

"This one creates its own light. And it is a good thing, too! We're going to see a lot and we need *lots* of good light for this one!"

The pages showed a field of dandelions basking in the sunlight. Thousands of yellow flowers upon a deep green canvas.

A single slender creek ran through the field of green and yellow, forming a sort of S-curve, or maybe like a stylized numeral "5."

Jenny held up the book to show her daughter, whose eyes grew wide and her smile—missing a tooth and all—grew even wider.

"That looks like such a nice place, Mom! Can we go there someday?"

Jenny grinned and put the book back in her lap. She turned the page with the creaking of thick, glossy paper and said, "Sweetie, we're going to go there right now! Just imagine the scent of the flowers...."

* * *

Jaina ran barefoot through the dandelion fields.

Soft grass and cold, moist dandelions comforted her feet as she ran, springing up again as she passed through.

Other flowers stood amid the dandelions but she loved them all equally. There were white flowers and pink and blue ones, all set against the deepest green grass, and the dandelions shone like droplets fallen from the sun on high.

The smell was so divine! Aromatic grass, wild and thick, met with the fragrances of sweet nectar.

Breathing it in was like feeling the soft petals gently caressing her face. Jaina could never get tired of it.

She knelt down and scooped a fuzzy white dandelion out of the earth. Holding it aloft, some of the seeds began to blow away on the wind.

Jaina watched them float, and she laughed because that was exactly what she wanted to wish for.

"I wish I could fly as you do, and see what you see!"

Then she pursed her lips and blew, scattering all but one seed from the dandelion head.

Before she moved on, she returned the plant to the ground and scooped dirt over its roots again.

The wind tugged at that last remaining parachute seed until it, too, floated away...right past Jaina's hand.

She reached out as if to catch it, and then she found herself swept up in the breeze.

The world swirled upward as she rose, hanging on to the dandelion seed, now grown to giant size.

No, wait, maybe she had shrunk so much that it was like a parachute carrying her across the meadow. Vivid colors blended into a living painting, stretching as far as the horizon.

Countless flowers waved in the breeze, each a little point of light, like a star in a deep emerald sky. About them wove beautiful music, thousands upon thousands of voices raised up together in song.

The wind whooshed and the dandelion seed soared as the ground fell away in rolling hills. She lifted higher into the sky, where winds flowed like river currents in an invisible ocean.

The sky darkened. Something passed by overhead, giving out a proud cry.

It was an eagle, soaring with its feathers in the sun. Jaina beamed as she looked up at it.

She had always loved birds, admired their freedom in flight, and now she has to experience the same thing.

The dandelion seed caught an updraft and higher she went still, hot on the tail of the mighty eagle.

Floating beside it, she laughed, and tears streamed from her face, in sheer joy.

This was something she had always wanted, and now her wish had come true!

The eagle looked over at her with a gleam in his golden eye. "Hello, stranger!" he said. "You wish to fly under the summer sun as I do?"

Jaina's heart leaped. "Yes! This is a wish come true, Mr. Eagle!"

The eagle's eyes turned back to the horizon. If it was possible, somehow a smile lifted the corners of his beak. "Then would you like to fly with me for a while? Just let go and I will bear you."

Jaina's eyes were round with awe. She looked up at the fluffy white dandelion seed.

"See you soon, okay? Don't forget me!"

And she let go, the seed obligingly floating along beside the eagle for a moment as he swooped lower and Jaina landed on his head.

Clinging to one feather, she shaded her eyes and found that she could see as the eagle saw.

Blue Mountains appeared out of what was a haze in the distance, rising and falling like distant waves.

Each flower she saw in clarity even from so high up, their petals glowing in the sun.
Trees rose like spires from the land, each holding an entire world in their branches.

The eagle saw all: the scurrying squirrels and the nesting birds, the hares and the deer, the fish gleaming in the far-away streams winding about the feet of the trees.

Here, this place was alive with the fullness of the summer, an inexhaustible flame of vitality.

Beyond the green and growing things, the eagle saw the spirits of land and sky, which frolicked as happily as a bird on the wing.

They were tiny like Jaina, or big like the eagle, sometimes both at once. Their lives mirrored that of the land itself.

Where they trod, life bloomed, and where life bloomed, they gravitated, forever finding meaning in the growth of the smallest seed, or the tranquility of the tallest tree.

Jaina realized that even during the day, when most were wide-awake and stretching out beneath the sun, the world dreamed, and she floated through its dreams at once an observer and a fellow traveler.

She breathed in deeply as the wind rushed across her face, granting her a sense of freedom she had never know before.
Here, sailing upon the sky itself, she knew what the golden days of late summer meant to all that lived within them.

She could feel the vibrant pulse of the world hot in her veins. It gave her such a sense of purpose, an invigoration that nothing else could match.

"You must not forget this feeling," said the eagle.

"This is life, my friend. Life at its purest. Enjoying sun, star, and moon. Breathing in the wind. Flying freely. You could weigh as much as a tree and still not burden me, for I am free. Here you are free, too."

A rocky outcropping stood tall over the bank of a wide blue lake below.

The eagle dipped his head. "Farewell, friend! Return whenever it pleases you!"

Jaina dove from the eagle's head turned and waved goodbye to him as she fell.

She spread her arms and let the wind slip through her fingers, cool and soft.

The lake grew as she fell toward it, but she was not afraid. Like a drop of rain, she broke the surface and plunged into another world.

The lake welcomed her as it welcomed the sunlight, which cast rays that soon became swirling mist within the waves.

And in the water's cold, refreshing embrace she saw more travelers. Big, silvery fish, their eyes bigger than her sprite-sized body, swam past, lazily enjoying the warm waters.

Jaina found that she could move through the water as freely as the eagle had the air, and she glided over to a bed of kelp that grew outward like a swaying forest.

A soft song like a hum rose from the kelp, celebrating its perspective: a green plant that enjoyed both water and sun in equal measure.

Jaina reached out and touched one of the leafy stalks and for a moment saw what the kelp saw: an entire kingdom stretching out across the bottom of the lake, and a sky ever shimmering at the surface.

Fish hid within its leafy mass. Crawdads crawled across the silt within its reach. Frogs and tadpoles danced to its endless tune. Ducks in the water sent ripples ringing like notes across the wave-sky above.

Pieces of driftwood floated by and some of the kelp would seize onto it, pulled free to drift with the wood.

The kelp saw all these lives bound together by the water and the growing earth and the sweet air above. Its perspective was truly blessed, to know so much of the lake's grand symphony.

Jaina swam back to the surface, buoyed by the haze of sunlight filtering down through the water.

She surfaced, listening to the plink and splash of the water.

Jaina lay back and closed her eyes, floating like a flower petal and simply enjoying the relaxing sounds.

She slept, or perhaps sleeping was the same as waking here, where dream and reality were one.

When she opened her eyes, no time had passed at all. The sun was still high in the sky above the lake, and a warmth rippled across the water.

Her breathing coincided with the rise and fall of the gentle waves. In, the water rose, lifting her toward the sky. Out, the water sank, and she felt cradled in a cool liquid bed.

In. Out. A year could have rolled past and she was so calm she would have never noticed it.

Presently a deep hum beat the air. Jaina opened her eyes.
A dragonfly hovered over the lake surface nearby, landing on a small piece of driftwood.

To the rest of the world, it was only a few inches long, but to Jaina the traveler, it looked to be closer in size to an actual dragon!

"Hello!" she called, waving. The dragonfly turned its head to her and its wings buzzed.

"Hello. Fine day, is it not?"

"Yes, it is!" Jaina clapped, incredibly amused that the dragonfly had answered her. "I have never enjoyed the lake so much."

The dragonfly buzzed in agreement. "Oh yes. The sun is pleasant and the water is refreshing. But I must be going. Will you need a lift?"

Jaina's eyes lit up.

"Could I?" She reached out, and the dragonfly lifted off, hovering over to her, and reached down one of its many hands to clasp hers.

Then the dragonfly laughed. "Do hold on!" With a humming *whoosh,* he was off and they flew above the lake, where leaves traveled on the wind and massive birds beat the air with their wings.

The dragonfly wove through it all skillfully, his wings ever humming like an endless guitar note.

Jaina looked down at the lake slowly strolling past beneath her, an amazing view of its shimmering surface from high up.

Never before had she had such a perfect wish granted?

A white cloud descended to fly next to her—no, not a cloud, the dandelion seed.

The very same one, she was sure of it.

"Thank you!" she called to the dragonfly before she let go and took hold of the floating seed again.

"May the winds bear you to wherever your heart desires!" called the dragonfly, and then he flew back down toward the lakeshore.

But Jaina floated upward and upward, the lake shrinking beneath her.

Soon she plunged into the clouds, rolling white mountains of mist and magic.

Jaina saw shapes therein: faces, animals, trees, castles. She saw glistening streams of water spiraling through the clouds like the dreams of rain. Cool moisture kissed her skin, warmed again by the sun when they emerged into the open blue air.

Jaina had never tasted such pure, sweet air, tinged with the scent of a fresh-fallen rain.

When the sunbeams hit the clouds just the right way they glittered like a field of stars.

Then one of the clouds would break and a torrent of rain fell, shining colors like stained glass as it poured down to the earth. Each raindrop was a different note and created the perfect symphony of sun and sky as she listened.

The dandelion seed passed through a wisp of cloud and Jaina, lulled nearly to sleep, let go.

She waved. "Farewell! Thank you for letting me fly with you!"

The seed floated slowly away, vanishing into the clouds, where its own dreams had always taken it.

Jaina lay back in a bed of pure softness, white like snow, warm like a lake in the sun, and clear as the air after a cleansing rainstorm. She spread her arms wide and closed her eyes.

A soft sound like the sighing of wind mingled with the gentle slosh of lake water filled all her mind.

Then she grew content, more so than she had ever known, freed as the wind and water, birds and clouds, from the burdens of her daily stresses.

Jaina slept in a sea of clouds and the smile never left her lips.

On a Mountain Top

From the mountain top, I look out and this is what I see
A tiny town, and a river running through the valley
Long wild grasses and multi-colored wildflowers grew all
around
I felt the heartbeat of the earth when I placed my hand upon
the ground

I could tell at once that this was some sort of scared space
And that my footprints should be the only thing I left in this
place
The birds sang from hidden spots in the ancient trees
Their song, grew more riveting as it was accompanied by the
bumblebees
Foxes played and yipped in the forest, hidden from view
Rabbits danced and jumped encircled in a field of bamboo

The old tribes called this place The Mountain of the Eagle
Trees, older than the oldest man reach to the sky, and stones
stand tall and regal
From this mountain top, I hear the voices of the generations
past
I know that I must preserve this hallowed spot so that it will
last

A Summer Night

The Air is full of expectation
The Sun burns hot in anticipation
Summer is close at hand
Natures fertility fills the land

Time for dancing and light
Sacred dancing through the night
Come jump over a fire
And wish for what it is that you desire

All fae folk gather in the wood
Singing "All of nature is good"
Frolicking upon the Earth Mother
Call her name Gaia or any other

Dance before the waterfall
Singing, dancing and merry-making one and all
Young faeries giggle under a flowering tree
A summer night; and all are free

The Lake

In the summer, the lake is my playground
In winter, I enjoy it when the tourists leave town
In spring, its surface is like reflective glass
In the autumn, the whitecapped waves crash

The lake is a place for fun and play
Or for celebrating Independence Day
The lake changes from season to season
I love it for this very reason
Living at the lake all of the time
Is, I must say, completely sublime
There is nothing quite like my little cabin on the lake
In every season, from heatwave to snowflake

The Dog Days of Summer

The dog days of summer are upon us
Heat radiates off every surface
The only relief is a lawn chair in the share
And a nice, tall glass of lemonade

A cooling breeze is nowhere to be found
Thank goodness, ice cream trucks abound
Playing their happy tune as they go along
Every kid in the neighborhood is chasing that song

The air is so hot and hazy
Such days as this were made for being lazy
A siesta, it seems is in part of the plan
Laying in the sun, getting a tan

Dandelion Journey

Once I took a journey upon a dandelion seed
In was the most magical ride indeed
First, I shrank until I was two inches tall
I grabbed ahold of a seed, a bit afraid of a fall

But soon I was aloft and riding the breeze
And away I went, as fanciful as you please
I traveled over many a meadow and field
And once by one, the secret places were revealed

I happened across a hidden butterfly glade
And watched as the fluttered in sunshine and shade
I hovered above the tree where the bees keep their hives
All of the workers, so busy to ensure their queen survives

And then I voyaged to the place where a young deer spent her
day
Secretly nestled in the tall grasses where her mother left her to
play
Watching over, in the branches of a tree, a bluebird did chatter
His eagle eye alerting the mother when something is the matter

And then, I arrived back at my home, all too soon
Back to normal, with the memories of a magical afternoon

If you ever get a chance to make a wish on a dandelion
Ask for a dandelion journey and soon you will be high flyin'

Cloud Gazing

Laying upon the summer grass, gazing into the clouds I see
A dog, a dinosaur and a 50-foot bumblebee
I have spent many a summer days
Staring into the sky, even though the late summer haze

The breeze blows and the hours pass me by
And still, I lay here looking up at the sky
Fluffy clouds tell stories one by one
From the first morning light until the day is done

Then comes in a strong breeze
That sends my clouds running, fast as you please
And when each marshmallow cloud has blown away
I shall smile remembering their playful display

Chapter 6: Autumn dreams

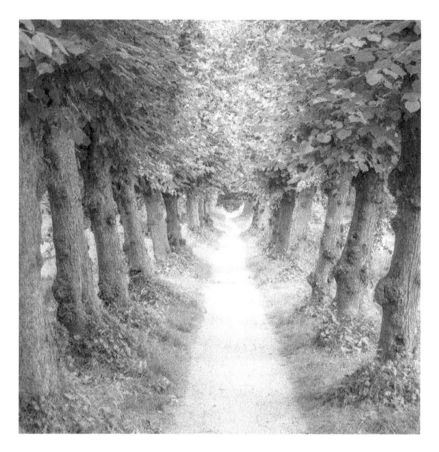

Jenny shook her head in dismay as she looked at her child, sitting amid a veritable pile of candy wrappers.

A cold Autumn breeze rolled in through the window and she got up to shut it.

"What am I going to do with you, kiddo? You are going to be up all night, bouncing off the walls with all that sugar! What was I thinking?"

Kirsty literally bounced on the bed, her gap-toothed grin fueled by entirely too much chocolate and marshmallow.

"Best Halloween ever, Mommy! I got, like, a hundred pounds of candy!"

Jenny laughed. The girl's enthusiasm was, if nothing else, infectious.
"I don't think quite that much, sweetie, but if you *did*, I'd box most of it up for next year!"

"Ewww!" Kirsty wrinkled her nose. "I don't wanna eat year-old candy!"

"I didn't say *you'd* have to eat it!" laughed Jenny.

"Maybe we'll give it to your father as punishment for letting you eat so much candy tonight!"

She sighed. Sometimes that man just did not think about things before jumping into them, and Jenny was left cleaning up the mess.

Kirsty giggled uncontrollably. "I bet he'd barf!"

"I'm sure."

"Do you think he would barf so much it'd fill up my candy bag, Mama?"

"Oh, gross, young lady! Let's not talk about such things before bed!"

Jenny reached out and lightly touched the tip of Kirsty's nose with her finger.

"Now, how am I ever going to get you to sleep in this condition? It's an impossible task!"

"What about a story, Mommy?"

Jenny put a finger to her lips and paused in thought.

"You know what? That's not a bad idea!"

She went to the self and picked up a well-worn paperback. "No, not that one!"

Jenny's fingers glided over to a thin storybook.

"Nope! The *big* one!"

Jenny picked up the heavy book with the crackling cover.

"Yes!"

As she sat on her daughter's bed, Kirsty managed to bounce even higher in anticipation.

"This book is the *best* one, Mommy! The stories in it really come to life! Better than the other ones."

"Okay, this one it is, sweetie. Now lay your head back and let me find a good one."

Though its covers were weathered, as Jenny slowly turned the pages to find the right story, they felt glossy and new as when she herself was a kid.

"Let me see, let me see...."

One chapter page stood out. A corridor of trees with leaves of red and gold arcing over a long road.

A lone branch had fallen in the road, a slender arm with a single thin shoot reaching away from the main branch.

It resembled a numeral "6," surrounded by falling leaves. As the mother and daughter watched, a few more leaves fluttered lightly to the ground.

"This is perfect for a brisk Autumn night. We have got a toasty fire going downstairs. If you listen, you can almost hear its warm crackle...."

* * *

Glimpses of a sunset through the trees sprawled red, orange, and purple across the Autumn sky.

The wind rustled the branches and fanned the leaves like crackling flames of red and gold that arced overhead.

Jaina felt as though she walked through a warm fire on the hearth itself.

The air was fresh but brisk with the Fall sweeping through, and alive with the energy of changing seasons.
She breathed in deeply and the air smelled of pumpkin patches, spiced apples, tree sap, and the wood fires burning.

This time of year had a special resonance as Summer gave way to Winter and the changes that swept in before the leaves fell.

Nights like tonight were magic. A living dream.

She almost needed no sleep; to walk down the street on such a night was as invigorating as any night's rest.

As Halloween approached, the world came to life with creatures and half-glimpsed spirits rarely seen outside of this time.

The change was upon the world, in the rich scents that wafted through the air of baking pies, of sweet apples upon the trees, of cold drafts from distant lands, and fires upon the hearth.
Smoke drifted from the chimneys as she passed rows of houses. Orange light shone warmly in the windows against the darkening world. The faded blue scarf she kept wrapped around her neck trailed behind her in the breeze.

There was a field at the end of the street that Jaina had loved since she was a child. It was fenced off now; full of tall grass, and the derelict structures she had played with was long gone.

An old rusted tractor. Concrete chunks left from a house demolished long ago. A small hill with an old well.

She had made up so many stories about the lives that went unfolded in that place, the staging site for her adventures into distant castles and faraway lands, or lazy summer naps with her friends while the butterflies flitted slowly overhead.

In Autumn, though, with a scarf around her neck and the change of seasons thick in the air, that field would serve as the gateway to many tales. As the butterflies changed through chrysalis, as the land changed during the Autumn, so did her stories involve metamorphosis.

Jaina walked through the gap in the fence, her fingertips trailing over the cold metal links.

A shiver ran through her as she crossed the threshold, but not because of the cold metal's touch; because she had stepped across the gateway and into another world.

The grass rose up around her steps, rippling in a sudden wind. Lights like fireflies appeared above trails that formed in the grass as hidden things scurried away.

A breath of wind spiraled around her, carrying with it leaves and memory: nutmeg and spice, a steaming hot cup of cocoa in the hands, smoke from the hearth fires, a soft but warm glow as the family huddled around the fireplace and shared stories. The perfect time of year.

Everything was transforming around her. Flowers opened in the field and then fell into slumber again.

Jaina knelt down, hearing a strange sort of symphony in the growth and decline of the flowers.

A hum, like an old playground song, or the music her mother would play as they all danced between kitchen and living room, preparing a celebratory feast as fiery-colored leaves carpeted the yard. And there!

Jaina turned and she saw an aged barrel sitting there in the grass amid a cloud of fireflies and butterflies. Water sloshed in the barrel and the smell of fresh apples filled the air.

The sound of laughter and children's voices followed, and then she saw them, as though they had just sprung from the tall grass.

One of the children was her. Some of them stood on stepstools made of logs. The older ones were tall enough to stand.

They took their turns bobbing for the apples, splashing each other with cold water, giggling like mad.

Leaves of yellow and red swirled about the outside of the scene, like a shifting wall between dream and waking worlds.

Jaina smiled, seeing her older sister push her head into the water before she was ready.

Young Jaina came up sputtering, a leaf sticking in her matted hair. She had been so furious with Melanie that day!

Looking back at it, she laughed. What she would give to go back to that time when her biggest worry was her siblings tormenting her!

Turning to her right, Jaina saw another wall of leaves before her, which parted as she approached.

This time she stepped into a scene she remembered all too well: the night of her thirteenth birthday party.

Jaina's whole family had gathered in the front room with Grandma Gail; that was the last birthday she would ever spend with her grandma.

The old woman smiled at her over her glasses, saving the best present for last. Jaina remembered it well: the very scarf she wore around her neck.

Grandma had knitted it herself over weeks, in Jaina's favorite color: a cool blue, like the Springtime morning sky.

She touched the fabric with her fingertips, still as soft as ever. Some of the colors had faded over ten years, but none of its comfort or warmth.

Grandma Gail had made it especially for those cooler Autumn nights that Jaina loved to explore.

Gail looked up and met Jaina's gaze with her kindly smile. Jaina's heart leaped. A breath caught in her throat.

She stood transfixed as Grandma Gail raised a hand and waved to her.

Of all sitting in the living room, only young Jaina noticed, and she turned her head, searching for whatever her dear grandmother saw.

Young Jaina shrugged and turned back to her scarf, holding it up in the firelight. She wrapped it around her neck and beamed a smile as Gail turned back to her.

Both of their eyes lit up as they shared a special moment that would make one of Jaina's favorite memories.

The leaves shifted again and Jaina found herself walking beside a creek in a forest. Late afternoon sunlight shone through a golden-red canopy.

She remembered the area well: she had walked here often as a child, and later would bring the young man who would one day become her husband on their first tentative date.

This time she was walking behind herself, as a young Jaina balanced precariously walking along a log fallen across the creek.

Older Jaina smiled, knowing what was coming. "Watch your step!" she called, and it seemed like her younger counterpart heard something through the mists of dream and memory.

She paused, but it was too late. Her foot slipped on moss and she tumbled into the creek with a splash.

The water was bitter cold. Jaina came up spluttering and gasping for air, shocked by the frigid water. She laughed and clambered out onto the shore.

Of course, she had to go back to dry off next to a fire in the backyard, but first, she saw what had caused her to slip: a small cocoon hanging on the knot where she was about to put her foot.

She had noticed it at the last second and trying to avoid it threw off her balance.

Young Jaina found that the timing was more blessed than cursed, however: the chrysalis was beginning to hatch.

A butterfly with drooping wings slowly crawled its way out of the cocoon, taking its first tentative steps as a young adult into an unsure world.

Jaina brushed dripping wet locks of hair from her eyes as she watched, shivering but fascinated.

The butterfly's wings slowly spread as it dried in the brisk Autumn air, patterned blue upon white, trimmed with black. A first few uncertain flaps tested the air.

Both Jainas watched with a bittersweet smile; both faced similar uncertainties, her younger self rapidly growing to meet the greater challenges of the world, and her older self-having struggled with those challenges.

Even now, she had to work hard and fight to make her own place in the world.

Yet here, in the dreams of Autumn, those burdens were laid aside. For like the butterfly, as it spread its wings with vigor and took to the sky, she had undergone her own metamorphosis.

From a girl to a young woman who had made her family proud, Jaina had learned to fly on her own as well.

She watched the butterfly as it fluttered up and around her, rising into the shafts of sunlight filtering down through the leaves. A trail of sparkling dust floated behind it like a river of tiny stars.

Jaina reached up and passed her hand through it, and when she drew it back, it seemed like she held for a moment a glimpse of the entire universe shining. Growth. Transition. Metamorphosis.

As the butterfly had undergone its many challenges to become who it was meant to be, so was she undergoing her own changes. Smiling, the older Jaina turned away. She remembered falling into the creek, but until now had forgotten what made her slip.

Now she felt that it was worth the cold and the discomfort to witness something so beautiful.

Her own thoughts rose with the wind like a fluttering leaf, whispering through the trees and into a starry evening sky.

Below her, the forest unfolded like a vast meadow of apple-red and sunshine-gold.

Ribbons wound through it in the form of the streams and creeks, helping to shape a vast tapestry.

The leaves would fall and carpet the ground in royal beauty, and the trees would stand naked in their beauty for a season.

Seeds slept in the earth's firm embrace, buds dreamed upon the branches. A blanket of frost covered all, turning to glisten dew in the morning sun.

Through it, all the land and all its dreaming creatures continued to grow and transform to find their Spring. For now, in Autumn's sweet embrace, the world slept and Jaina floated above it in peaceful memory.

In the Autumn of the Year

In the Autumn of the year
When a brisk wind is what I hear
A cup of cocoa awaits

As the leaves, fall one by one
I am relieved that the day is done
All of my stress abates

I put my tired feet up
And reach for my favorite cup
While reaching for my favorite book

As the fire burns low
And the candles star to lose their glow
I give the room one last look
And then it is off to bed
I close my eyes and rest my weary head
Hoping that dreams find me fast

As I sleep, the night wears on
And pushes towards a misty dawn
It is the Autumn of the year, at last

The Rosebud

She is the beginning of a stunning flower
A delicate rosebud awaiting the coming hour
There in the shadows, just on the verge
She is a beautiful rose, waiting to emerge

Ever reaching for her place the sunlight
Beautiful flower wait until the time is right
Feeling so small and unnoticed, it seems
Little rosebud be patient to wait for your dreams

Your time as a rosebud pass by fast
And soon your bloom will come at last
You will open then, full of beauty and grace
And as the star of the garden take your place

,

All will stop and in wonder, they will stare
At you, the beautiful rose growing there
Feel your inner beauty, my little friend
And know that it will burst forth in the end

Fall

My favorite time of year is fall
Pumpkin spice everything, bonfires, and football
Leaves are turning orange, gold, and red
And the sun goes earlier each night to his bed

Drinking coffee and watching the frosty dawn
And watching the deer play, a mother and last year's fawn
Reading a book by a cozy fire
Remembering all the things to which I aspire

I light an apple-scented candle
And grab my teacup by its delicate handle
I settle in for a much-needed restful day
Yes, Fall is my favorite time of year all the way

Emergence

He is emerging from a cocoon
More than just a caterpillar,
He will be a butterfly soon

He struggles, and he tries
To strengthen his wings
He must work before he flies

Filled with frustration and doubt
Sure, that he will not make it
He fears he will never get out

But future before him is bright
He is wonderful and amazing,
And soon he will take flight

When his emergence is complete
We will all cheer his success
As he flies away without defeat

Summer's End

Now is the time of Summer's End
Not as much, free time to spend
Summer tourist have all gone home
And I walk the lakeshore alone

Time to say goodbye to those days so warm and lazy
Now everything is going to be fast and crazy
Time for bonfires and jumping in piles of leaves
Drinking hot cocoa, and wearing long sleeves

I anticipate the cooler, shorter days
Yet, I miss basking in the sun's rays
It happened so fast, I can hardly remember
Yesterday it seemed, was June, and now it's September

As I light Autumn's first cozy fire,
My cocoa in hand, almost ready to retire
I reflect up the season just passed
Smiling at the memories of love and laughter, always to last

Autumn's Call

Though summer's heat lingers still
I can hear Autumn's call
With anticipations, I long for its chill

I await the leaves of red and gold
And hot apple cider
To chase away the cold

I am ready for pumpkin spice
Bonfires and bobbing for apples
And a hayride would be nice

The end of summer is near
In the hot, hazy afternoon
Autumn's call is all I hear

Autumn

The days grow short and the leaves are turning
The chill creeps in while bonfires are burning.
Autumn has arrived at long last
Riding in with skies, cloudy and overcast

In every window, Jack o' Lanterns are glowing
And the season's first flurries are snowing
Pumpkin pies are in the oven baking
And candy is set out, free for the taking

Hot cocoa with marshmallows fills every mug
And spiced apple cider is made by the jug
Families and friends are all gathered together
Drawn closer by the cold, rainy weather.

Autumn is by far the coziest time of year
So many stories to tell and to hear
Then snuggle under the blankets for the long night
And let all of your Autumn dreams take flight

Chapter 7: Winter dreams

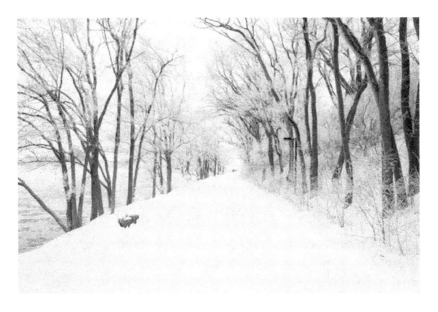

Jenny watched as the snow continued to fall and mount outside the window.

Fog lightly obscured the window.

She reached up to rub some of it away, her fingers squeaking on the cold glass.

A steaming mug of hot cocoa warmed her hands, and she curled her fingers around the warm mug. Another mug sat on the windowsill beside her.

The lights were low in the living room, except for the fireplace, which crackled with a merry fire. Shadows danced across the room.

Kirsty lay on the floor in front of the fire, resting her chin in her hands, watching the shapes that formed and melted away just as quickly in the flames.

Soft holiday music played on a speaker.

Kirsty hummed along with it.

The snow finally started to slow. Larger flakes fell lazily upon a city blanketed in white.

The steady sound of a snow shovel scraping on the driveway kept Jenny's thoughts occupied.

Her husband was out there shoveling. It was only snow, but it was cold enough that she worried.

At last, the scraping sounds stopped, and the snowfall dwindled to nearly nothing.

The front door opened and a tall man with a scarf around his neck, a white-flecked wool hat, and very red cheeks stepped in.

Jenny picked up the cup of cocoa and went to meet him at the door.

She helped him get his coat, hat, and scarf off, and then handed him the mug.

"Welcome back, hon. Looks like it's finally stopped."

He took the mug and sipped slowly from it, blowing wisps of steam away.

"Oh, you always make the best cocoa, babe. How do you do that? I can never get it as good as yours!"

He went out to the living room and sat on the floor near Kirsty, who also had some cocoa—though the girls were maybe more marshmallow than cocoa at this point!

Jenny retrieved her own cup and joined them.

"At least it wasn't too bad, this time. Not like last year!"

"Last year was awesome!" Kirsty exclaimed.
Jenny laughed. "Oh, no, my dear. It was not! We were snowed under for two days! Don't you remember when your father broke the snow shovel? We couldn't do anything!"

"Nuh-uh, Mommy! Remember how I tunneled out of the downstairs bathroom window?"

"Don't you *ever* do anything like that again! That was dangerous!"

Despite herself, Jenny smiled. The girl was certainly irrepressible. Snow, rain, none of it slowed her down.

However, the last winter had been pretty concerning, so Jenny made sure to stock up on firewood and candles.

Her husband stood up and went out the back sliding door to go retrieve more firewood.

Jenny had an idea. "Why don't we do a family story night, in front of the fire? Would you like that, sweetie?"

"YES!" The girl's shriek of affirmation could have caused an avalanche!

"Okay, baby, but keep it down! Your sister is asleep. Let me go get the book."

Jenny stood up and slipped out of the room, heading back through the living room to the stairs. She had left the storybook up in Kirsty's room.

While she was upstairs, she stopped to check on the baby; the monitor was quiet, but she just wanted to be sure. The baby girl was asleep and looked happy and peaceful.

Jenny smiled and went back downstairs.

Kirsty was sitting up now, excitedly rocking back and forth while her father piled up wood near the fireplace.

She begged him to let her put in the next one, and he handed her a piece of chopped wood.

Kirsty zealously tossed it into the fire, leaving her father to hurry and maneuver it into an optimal place with the firepower. That done, they both sat back, their faces aglow in the firelight. Kirsty came and sat next to them, all sharing one big blanket, sitting back against the front of the couch. She set the book down on her lap.

"Okay, you two." Jenny smiled knowingly.

"I think I have the perfect story for this kind of night."

She opened the book and flipped to a page showing a beautiful snow-covered landscape.

Peaks of purest white rose into a pale blue sky.

The plains of snow that spread across the page glowed with cool white light, filling the living room, mingling with the golden firelight above their heads like an aurora.

In the ice a crack had formed, taking the shape of a numeral "7."

"This one is going to take us to someplace that'll look a little familiar right now...."

* * *

A biting wind blew across the vast plains of glittering white.

Dusty snow stirred on the surface layer. Huge drifts had built up over months and formed a hilly terrain of round white hills, jagged peaks, and smoothly blanketed valleys.

Here and there, the tundra peeked through the snow, dark green mottled spots against the bluish-white scenery. Even as the sun shone down, the snow and ice sparkled as though studded with diamonds. It was cold but beautiful beyond measure.

Jaina stood at the top of a small ridge and shaded her eyes. She wrapped the scarf around her neck and smiled.

What a view it was!

So comparable to the snow-covered cars, driveways, and yards she had seen before she went to bed, having shoveled the driveway for the third time that day.

This was an amazing view, and she would never dream of marring it with backbreaking shoveling. Nor could even a giant shovel all the snow of this place.

Her boots crunched in the snow as she walked.

Her breath steamed in the air, curling away in wispy fingers.

The cold reddened her skin but did not harm her; she walked among the land, as did a traveler through a dream: present but ethereal, safely experiencing another world.

She could breathe in deeply and feel the ache in her lungs from the cold, dry air, and yet it did not hurt. Rather, it added a sense of life to the setting, gave her a greater feeling of immersion in the blindingly bright arctic lands.

To untrained eyes, the place looked barren, but those who could see beyond the surface saw an entire world of life.

Tufts of green shrubs and thick carpets of lichen and moss-covered much of the ground.

Snow piled in and around the greenery, but there was always something growing through, even in the coldest parts. More things grew in the tundra. A

family of white-furred hares peeked their heads up over one of the snow dunes. They seemed to notice Jaina but did not mind, rather chittering excitedly among themselves.

They had found some food and shared it together as a family: two adult hares and two younger ones. Their fur was so soft and fluffy it could have been made of fresh-fallen snow in itself.

Once they had finished eating, as a family they all bounded away, soon disappearing into a burrow made into the snow berms. They nestled down in their cozy den to enjoy the rest of the day.

Jaina hopped along, feeling as carefree and light-footed as a hare.

It was hard not to feel the light-hearted spirit of the happy little creatures in such a bright and beautiful land.

She came to a chasm, where snow looked over cliffs of a pale, luminous blue ice.

The wind whistled and howled through the chasm.

Her footstep disturbed a pile of snow, which tumbled down into the blue abyss, and she smiled. Its mysteries called to her.

She could not resist the temptation to take a look.

When Jaina stepped down, her own reflection in the ice fractured into a thousand different images, each one grinning back at her as she drifted downward light as a snowflake.

The ice walls seemed to hold mysteries of their own frozen dream-shapes and glimpses as through a lens into distant worlds.

One object half-hidden in the thick ice could have been an elephant-like creature, still locked in its icy dreams since ages past.
Jaina reached out and touched the ice over it, and suddenly she found herself transported to an ancient yet familiar land.

The giant furred beast walked as the king of the land, unchallenged in its pride and power.

Tundra spread out before it, but as the warmer months had caused some of the ice to recede, a vast realm of green and yellow sprawled across the horizon.

Ice formed peaks and capped hills, but the land was very much growing even amid all the ice and snow.

Hares leaped from dune to dune, becoming part of the snow for brief moments as they vanished into the flaky puffs.

Snow owls flew over the snow, their feathers impossibly bright, like shafts of pure light radiating from their wings.

Jaina watched in fascination as they flew past, their round eyes like miniature suns, shining beams before their path.

She wanted to reach out but they were too fast and too high for her to reach, even as the giant.
Still, all fled her path as she walked from sunrise to sunset, and then hunkered down to sleep the night away....

Jaina drifted away from the frozen giant, smiling. She had gotten to take part in his dreams and loved every second of it.

However, her own called. Jaina floated upward, rising with a sudden updraft out of the chasm, buoyed by the crisp arctic air. She spread her arms wide and spun as she lifted up, spiraling up into the sunlight.

There was so much more to see and do in such a place, this endlessly breathtaking land of snow and wonder.

A shrill, piping cry greeted her as she noticed a herd of caribou thundering past.

They sang as they ran together, a song of unity and hope, always excited for what lay over the next hill, just over the next horizon.

They were a family, shaggy-coated and covered in frost, but they were always there for one another. As the herd ran, they jostled and shifted positions, with the young in the middle of the herd.

Each raised their voice up as they came to their new position. So too did their footsteps and their snorting breaths add to the greater music of the arctic wonderland.

For a time Jaina ran with them, her feet gracefully skimming the top of the snow.

She felt what it was like to belong to the herd, be part of a big family, out there in the open tundra.

Sometimes, they had only each other to rely on for warmth, support, companionship, and as part of that, Jaina felt a sense of camaraderie she had rarely experienced.
She felt stronger to be part of the herd, each one helping to keep the others running lightly and happily.

Their dreams were that of the land itself: of endless plains of white and green, enough food to fill every belly in the herd, and a starry sky at night to guide their slumber.
They welcomed the moon as much as they did sun, and they enjoyed the bounties that the land gave freely. Theirs was a rugged existence, simple, a family together in the beautiful northern wilderness.

Jaina bid them farewell and ran on, as they turned away and ran eastward.

She saw that the land soon gave way to a shelf and beyond it the frigid but alluring arctic waters.

Jaina stooped and dipped her fingers into the crystalline water, sending out a series of ripples that each rang with a high, clear note.

All at once, the entire arctic sea came to life with the same music, each crest and splash like a ringing instrument playing a sweet tune.

Far out from the ice-locked shore a great shape emerged from the water. It gleamed black as onyx, with great white spots upon its head and a belly white as snow. Jaina cheered as more appeared.

They were orcas, one of her favorite kinds of animals. A big family of them all journeying together with the currents.

One by one as they surfaced each spouted, and the spouts rose like mists of many colors, and a haunting song played as the droplets rained back down to the surface again.

The pod of orcas arced gracefully through the waves, the ripples they sent out joining with the ones Jaina had created.
Then the whales dove and vanished again into the cold waters, and Jaina wanted more than anything to follow them did.

The sun began to sink and she hopped out onto the ice floes, springing lightly from one to the other, hoping to catch another glimpse of the orcas.

The wake of their passage left an easy trail, but Jaina could not seem to keep up with them. There! One breached the surface not too far away from the floes as if to show her they were nearby.

The waves cast by its huge body impacting sent the ice floes bobbing unsteadily and Jaina stepped off into the cold waters. Downward she plunged in a cloud of bubbles, her bright eyes seeking a glimpse of that which she loved.

She swam easily, as though floating through the air itself, and found herself faced with the most magnificent sight she had ever seen.

Rays of faint light splayed down from the shimmering surface.

In the flowing currents deeper down the light became as clouds of luminous mist. She dove further down, following the orcas, who in the dim and refracting light appeared to be made of the night sky itself.

The light became undulating ribbons of many colors, stretched across a vast sky that rolled like ocean waves.

Tiny pinpoints of brightest white appeared in the surface and she realized that she swam among the orcas through an ocean of stars.

Here, as the northern lights filled the heavens with their mysterious glow, the borders between sea and sky had vanished completely.

The orcas were vessels filled with the stars, and so were her eyes. They flew as one into the aurora and the sounds of their joyful, haunting songs blended with Jaina's laughter.

Ripples of their harmony spread across the aurora, which danced all through the night.

Jaina and the pod of orcas drifted through the atmospheric orchestra as conductors and listeners alike.

She became enveloped in the ethereal colors: green and pale blue, even red.

The sky was aflame with pure light, a place where the dreaming mind was the truth and the waking world was dispelled by the song of the world itself.

Jaina had never known such bliss as she let go all of her worries and became one with a piece of music as old as the planet itself.

The orcas flew about her, leaping, spinning, and drifting along with her. To them, this was the night sky lit by the aurora as they experienced it, but Jaina was new to such a perspective.

Now that she had known it, she could never sleep the same way again.

Great notes formed in the aurora, carrying the sleeping night through and welcoming the coming dawn.

Jaina and her fellow dreamers slept soundly in the sky, held aloft by the most ancient and primal of songs.

Nothing could disturb their rest, as they became another part of the grandest composition.

All who looked up and saw the aurora found their hopes and dreams buoyed the same way, moved to float amid a cosmic chorus from which one could only know peace.

The Faeries' Winter Night

On a silvery, misty, moonlit night.
Winter faeries dance with delight

Frost flakes forming fast.
On every flower and blade of grass

The night so cold yet not still.
Dancing faster now coming up from inside the hill.

White and silver and dazzling blue
Come to celebrate when the winter is new

Dancing slows as the night wears on
One by one, Winter faeries yawn

Eyes so heavy, they yearn to close.
Returning now to the hill, seeking repose.

Changing Seasons

The seasons are changing
And everything is rearranging
Summer's end is fast approaching
And Autumn's winds are encroaching

Summer holds trying to last a bit longer
But Autumn's chill grows stronger
The eternal struggle that is forever repeated
Summer always trying, always defeated

Autumn, don't be so smug at Summer's abating
Don't, you know at your end Winter is waiting.
So, enjoy your season while it lasts
For soon comes, the Winter's icy blasts

First Snowfall

I look out the window in anticipation
The weatherman has promised frozen precipitation
This will be the day of the first snowfall
It will bring joy to once and all

As the first flurries fly
The children will run outside with a glad cry
They will catch snowflakes on their tongue
Before you know it, a winter song was sung

When the snow begins to stick
Everyone will get their sleds and be extra quick
Racing to the bottom of the hill
Everyone squeals as they take a spill

Finally, everyone comes in to warm by the fire
And get ready for the night and time to retire
One last cup of cocoa and then it is off to bed
I'll tuck you in, hear your prayers and kiss you on the forehead

Faces in the Firelight

Look closely and you will see faces in the firelight
They're dancing in the middle is a fire sprite
She spins and twirls and giggles with delight

Look closer and you will see so many more
Faces of those who have gone on before
So many mysteries in the fire to explore

Chapter 8: The desert

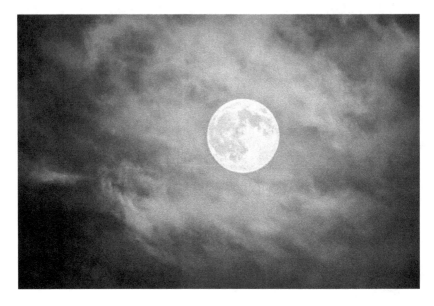

Jenny stuck her face out the window, letting the brisk night air roll over her, whipping her hair back.

The kids were asleep.

The car was quiet, and the only sound in the night was the sound of the tires rolling sibilantly along the road.

Her husband drove so she could relax, and though sleep tugged at her eyelids, she wanted to stay awake a little longer.

They were headed out on vacation, which meant a drive across the desert, and she loved the desert. It was always so peaceful, and as a child, her parents had often taken them out in the RV into the desert to experience a little bit of camping outside of the usual spots.

The desert at night was one of the most incredibly beautiful places Jenny had known in her life.

A deep blue sky twinkling with stars blanketed the land, flat but for the buttes that occasionally rose up in the distance.

Cacti stood tall, their spiny arms raised, the moving shadows making them appear as if waving at the passing car.

Deep shadows pooled in the small ravines and gullies as they drove past.

Night birds gave their hooting cries, and the steady chirp of crickets made Jenny drowsy.
Her head nodded once, then twice. She yawned so hard that tears started in her eyes.
Jenny tried to shake away the sleepiness but her eyelids remained heavy.

Blinking through the fatigue, she thought that the full moon looked a little funny.

Clouds had passed in front of its center, making it resemble a giant yellow number "8."

At last, she laid her head back against the seat and let the wind rushing through the open window soothe her.

She closed her eyes and soon her dreams wandered into the desert night.

Just like one of the stories in her book....

* * *

A young Jaina stepped out of the family camper and into the clear night.

The sky was a vast night blue canvas upon which trails of stars were painted.

A pale light loomed on the horizon as the sunset faded from the sky.

She loved the nights out here, camping where you could hear the coyotes and the crickets.

No sound of cars, no doors slamming, no machines rattling. Only the soft whoosh of the open air and the sounds of the creatures that lived in the desert.

Jaina liked to pretend she was one sometimes. She wondered what it would be like to live like the desert birds or the mice or even the snakes and lizards.

Jaina imagined a little kangaroo mouse, like the kind she had seen last night on the edge of the firelight. Her gaze wandered across the hundreds of little paths and hiding places visible in the light of the fire.

She knew better than to wander too far and disturb a sleeping stinger of some kind, but here, in the little ring of rocks and cacti where they had parked the camper, she was safe to explore.

Elsewhere, a mouse tentatively hopped out of its little burrow—to the mouse, it was a cave, but to the world outside, it was barely a hole. For a young kangaroo mouse, it was the only home she needed.

As the night fell dark and chilly upon the desert, she was on a mission: to simply enjoy the night. On other nights, she might seek out food, or friends, but tonight was more like a journey through the dreams of the desert itself.

She might have been a traveler, safely asleep in her den, or perhaps blessed enough to feel part of another dreamer's adventure.

When the lines between worlds blurred, story and reality were not so different, after all.

Tonight, she was safe to explore.

Her burrow opened out onto a dried-up riverbed. It had been many long months since water coursed down the channel, and it would not tonight, but the land itself remembered the taste.

The mouse did not need the water to survive. To her, it was a strange and wondrous occurrence when the skies opened up and poured cold drops upon the desert.

Then the waterways would run like torrents and she would have to hide in a nice, cozy, dry burrow.

Smooth rocks and dusty shrubs currently filled the riverbed. Deep shadows enshrouded them. A single cricket stood atop a nearby rock and belted out its high-pitched night song.

The mouse stopped and the looked at it.

"Beautiful night for music," said the mouse.

"Music is for every night!" said the cricket, and he stopped playing long enough to answer her.

"The night, she sings to me. Does she sing to you?"

"I only hear your song," said the mouse. "But I feel like there is more out there tonight, so I am going to find it."

"Then I wish you luck!" And the cricket began to play again, this time a song of exploration and discovery.

The hopeful tune accompanied the mouse as she bounded down the riverbed from perch to perch.

Tall rocks like cliffs overlooked the path, littered with dust and spotted with tough little shrubs and weeds.

The tracks of other nocturnal creatures also formed trails in the sun-baked terrain.

The mouse recognized many of them: snakes, lizards, desert tarantulas, and her own trails from past nights.

Each was a snapshot of life in the desert. To outsiders, the land seemed arid and barren, barely able to sustain life.

As the mouse journeyed through this very vibrant world, it was all very much alive with an entire world hidden in the stones and sand.

A constant cacophony of bird whistles filled the air, alternating like the creaking metal joints of a wheel.

Hidden just behind a line of rocks, some insect crawled with a sibilant scratch. It was a huge black beetle, gleaming in the night, its antlers on proud display as it thrust one of the rocks, bigger than its own body, aside to make a path.

"Oh. Good. Evening." The beetle spoke in a very slow and plodding monotone.

"You are very strong!" said the mouse, her own voice excited. She had never seen such a beetle before and found him endlessly fascinating.

"Oh. Maybe. I. Am." The beetle crawled slowly into the riverbed, now becoming a highway for the passage of the desert's many living creatures as the sunset faded and night deepened. "But. You. Are. Very. Fast!" The beetle turned and began to crawl in the direction the mouse had come from.

"If you need a place to stay for the night, please use my burrow! I won't be back until the morning!"

The mouse wanted to be charitable. She had never seen anything like this beetle and was hoping to meet him again, but she could not stay. Adventure called!

"Thank. You." The beetle stopped and turned his great horned head. "Maybe. I. Will!"

"You are welcome!" The mouse squeaked with delight and bounded down the path again.

A bird sleeping in the arm of a cactus overlooking the path awoke as she paused and looked down at her.

It was a wren, brown, white, and fluffy, like the mouse. It waved its wings at her and then tucked its head into sleep again.

But the mouse felt fortunate. The wren's feathers reminded her of her family, and it made her all the more excited to see them again.

Many shapes loomed up out of the dark. The cacti were as towers, but in the shrubs, a warm wind rustled.

The mouse felt as though she ran into a forest, which moved endlessly as she turned a bend in the riverbed.

The banks were much higher here when in days past the river had rushed through with greater strength.

Long ago, the voice of those waters had filled the land, and all who came to this little valley would hear them.

For the song of the river was a timeless one, at once ancient and yet eternally young.

Always changing, but always retaining the same purpose in life.

The little mouse climbed the steep banks, hopping from purchase to purchase, until at last, she scrabbled up to the very top, to her a bluff overlooking a mighty riverbed.

There she saw the channel that the water had once delved into the land itself and she wondered what it must have been like, back when the desert's dreams were full of water.

As if in answer to her desire, a sudden rumbling in the earth accompanied a liquid roar.

The mouse looked up the slope of the riverbed and saw it coming, a torrent of silvery water that rolled forth with a clamor.

In the foam and spray as it came, shapes of the desert formed and then melted away just as quickly, each an embodiment of the lives that the river touched.

A great spider appeared upon a web of water droplets and then blended into a clutch of newly hatched snakes experiencing their first taste of the warming sun.

The curious snakes dove into the waves and up emerged owls with wings spread wide, and eyes like lamps.

The owls flapped their splashing wings and became bats, sending out a song that echoed through the water.

When the bats dropped back to the water out sprang hares and bighorn sheep, and behind them leaping deer and laughing foxes.

The river rushed past, and as it came, the very air shimmered and seemed to change.

A smell of ozone followed.

Thunder crackled in the sky far above.

Rain fell, eager to join the river on its course through the dusty flatlands.

All at once, as if awoken from slumber, countless voices rose in a murmur at the rain's sweet song.

This was one of the miracles of the desert, an occurrence so rare that the parched earth scarcely recalled the taste of water.

Now the little kangaroo mouse got to witness what it had always dreamed of—and it was truly beyond imagination.

One of the wrens landed on the outcropping beside her and shook its rain-soaked feathers.

"So lovely!" he said in a loud voice belying his little size, not much bigger than the mouse herself.

"What a night to be alive! It is said that often the desert dreams of the rain, but rarely do the dreams come true."

He turned to the mouse. "Good evening, friend! Do you come here to see the river, too?"

The mouse hopped excitedly up and down. "I wanted to see what this place was like when the great water was still here! And now I can! But is this real or are we seeing the past?"

The wren laughed in answer. "Friend that is the wrong question to ask!"

"What is the right question?" the little mouse said, eager to know the answers she sought. But the cagey old wren only laughed again.

"The question is not what *is*, or *was*, or what *will be*. The question is simply: what does this mean to *now*?"

Despite her best attempts, the young mouse simply could not understand. "What do you mean, Mr. Wren? I don't understand that, either!"

The bird lifted his wings and spread them wide. "Because you are young, and you seek out the purpose of the dream. You look for what course the river runs to understand it, but that is not the river's way. The river flows upon whatever course awaits it. The river does not question why it simply experiences the thrill of its adventure."

"Am I not to question, then?" The little mouse felt dejected, but soon the wren lifted her spirits again.

"You should always question! Always seek the truth behind the dream. What you must learn one day is that sometimes the dream is the truth itself, and the truth is the dream. Can one exist without the other? Do you feel the water, hear its voice, and bask in its embrace? Yes? Then the river is real, whatever its origin or path."

With that, the wren bid her goodnight and flew off into the rain, whistling loudly and cheerfully.

The little mouse clapped her paws and watched as the river rushed past, telling the story of the desert's history and foretelling its future.

Year by year, she returned to that spot to experience the same dream, and year by year, she grew to understand what the old wren had meant.

One day she became a mother and a grandmother and patriarch to a large and thriving mouse family, and still, she came back to that spot, long after the wren had gone.

One day, she stood there as the river crashed through, and another young mouse climbed up to that very same hill.

His little eyes grew wide as he observed the momentous event; overcome with the magic of the waters he had seldom known. And he asked the very same question that the little kangaroo mouse had once asked of the wren.

"I have never seen anything like this! Is this real?"

The old kangaroo mouse smiled.

* * *

Jaina awoke with a yawn. She had not even realized that she had fallen asleep until she felt the first few raindrops on her skin.

The fire had died down, but there was a curious little mouse standing near it.

Jaina smiled and started to reach out to it but the mouse hopped away...though not out of fear.

It jumped for the sheer joy of the desert night. As she watched it go, Jaina felt like she had known a little of what that was like.

Then a bird atop the camper called to her, a little brown wren before it flew off into the night as well.

Jaina watched it go as the rain began to fall drop by drop.

She heard the songs of the crickets and the cicadas, and in the distance, a coyote howled to greet the rain.

Even the fire, sizzling as it was with each drop, seemed to be sighing in relief at the welcome return of an old friend.

She looked up into the stars and breathed in the sweet smell of fresh rain, the tang of parched dust soaking up the moisture, and the cool caress of the breeze.

Long after Jaina went back inside the camper that night, she dreamed of dusty plains, rivers rushing, and mice hopping freely.

As the night passed and the sky began to lighten again, an old kangaroo mouse hopped into the campsite. She stared at the camper curiously for a long moment.

"I wonder what they are dreaming?" the mouse said to herself.

Then she had a strange feeling that she already knew, and the thought brought her peace. With the sun coming up, it was time for her to return to the burrow where food, slumber, and family awaited.

She hopped away, content in sharing her desert dreams with all the others in her blessed home.

As she neared her burrow, the old mouse heard the cry of a wren.

Then, in the distance, she thought she heard the whoosh and burble of rushing waters.

She smiled and closed the door to listen to the water while she slept.

Water Gazing

Sitting and watching the river flow
Wondering where it is that it will go
Never to tarry at the same place
Always a forward-moving race

I cast my troubles and cares to the river
I watch the eddies and currents until I shiver
Water, it washes all my strife away
And to it, I return to play

Desert Night

The heat of the day has gone at last
And the cool midnight blankets this land, so vast
Some might see this panorama as desolate and bare
But if you look, life is thriving everywhere

The coyote howls in the distance of the night
Under a desert sky, no moon but stars are bright
A mouse scurries from his home, in search of a meal
Avoiding the night predators, he has nerves of steel

In a saguaro cactus silhouetted in the dark
Is the hidden home, of a sleeping little lark
An owl hoots somewhere up in the blackened skies
Searching for the prey that will not escape his sharp eyes

The desert night has a multitude of surprises to behold
It can only be witnessed by those who are bold
Look closely and it's secrets it shall reveal
The desert night, such mysterious appeal

Sunrise on the Horizon

The sun wakes up from his slumber and begins his accent
As the moon maiden finishes her early morning decent
The sunrise on the horizon in a magnificent sight
First, pinks and then oranges and then the yellow so bright

Sunrise over the ocean, one of nature's treasures
Watching it every morning is one of life's simple pleasures
The earth warms under his nurturing rays
Waves reflect his light back in awesome displays

Sunrise it the most perfect time of day
Everything is fresh and new and ready for work or play.
Nothing is better than basking in the light of the newly born
sun
When the day has just begun

Desert Skies

Into the desert night, we walk, hand in hand
Gently we place a blanket upon the sand
Cacti dot the landscape making up nature's skyline
Here in the desert, barrenness and life combine

Millions of stars are close enough to touch
We spot the big dipper, and Orion and such
A shooting start tears a path of light
And I make a wish that we could live forever in this night

I am surprised by the unexpected chill in the air
The daytime had been so hot, I must compare
Suddenly another meteor makes its way to the ground
And soon falling stars are all around

The desert sky is a magical sight to behold
I know we will still come to watch, even when we have grown
old
Here we are surrounded by the beautiful rugged charm
Then with the sunrise, we leave arm in arm.

The Moon

I see the moon rising above the mountain top
The night sky is illuminated with her magic
Clouds drift slowly by, but her light will not stop
Higher she travels in the sky
Watching everyone from her vantage point
As the long, lovely night passes by

Lady Luna shine your moonbeams down
Fill my soul with laughter
And spread happiness and peace throughout the town

Now I watch as the moon sets into the sea
Gone to bed for the day
But I smile knowing that tonight she will return to me.

Chapter 9: A cosmic highway of dreams

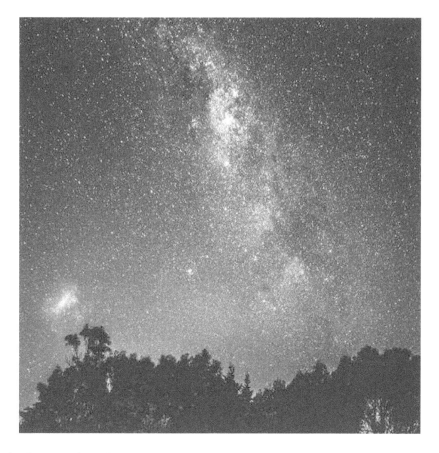

The last night of their camping excursion dawned and Jenny sat with her daughters out in the cool night air.

She breathed deeply. The scent of recent rain was sweet.

Nearby, the lake waves reflected the last rays of the setting sun into a golden sheen.

Everything felt washed clean and refreshed. Evergreen trees towered over the campsites, giving off the tangy aroma of pine sap.

A few birds still hooted and chirped in the trees, but one by one, they were dropping off into silence, leaving the crackling and popping fire to mingle with the soft lake sounds.

Jenny sat in a camping chair by the fire, holding her youngest to her chest.
Kirsty sat in the chair beside her, hugging a blanket around herself. The orange firelight danced upon their features.

Stars appeared in the sky overhead, white gems set upon a blue tapestry.

Jenny craned her head back to look up at them, and Kirsty followed suit.

Some stars shone brighter than others did, some were steady, and some flickered rapidly. The view was enchanting. At last Kirsty spoke.

"Mommy, do you ever wonder what's out there?"

"All the time, sweetie. I used to dream of it quite a lot. I wanted to be an astronaut when I was your age. I still think it'd be amazing to go out there and explore someday."

"I wanna be an astronaut, Mommy! Could I?"

"Baby, you know we've always told you to just follow your dreams. If you want to be an astronaut and see the stars or an astrophysicist and see what makes them work, you should do that."

"But what if I want to see what the stars dream, Mom? Do you think the stars and planets dream like that?"

Jenny smiled. "Well, then I suppose you'd be an artist, hon. Poets, painters, writers, performers, they've all been inspired at times by the view from down here. I used to paint some when I was a kid, too. I used to know the trick to making the paintings really come to life!"

"Aww, I'll bet you could still do it, Mommy! Just like your book!"

At that, Jenny grinned knowingly. "You mean this book, dear? This one right here?"
She lifted the heavy book and opened it to one of the last chapters.

"You asked what it was like to become a dreamer of the stars. Well, let me show you a small piece of that place. It's pretty amazing...."

The picture that graced the page was a galaxy spinning in a milky torrent of stars.

Beyond it, one could see vast nebulas and cosmic pathways leading to the ineffable mysteries of the universe.

But the stars shone so brightly that for a moment before Jenny turned the page, night turned to day within the endless night of space itself.

Kirsty gasped, and then her mother turned the page....

* * *

Jaina leaned her head against the window as the miles rolled past.

Back through the desert, where things were open and quiet, back home to the city.

She would be glad to be home but it was hard to leave such beauty behind.

As she looked up, she saw one particular star twinkle ever brighter.

It seemed to beckon her gaze and her flight of fancy. She wondered at its impossibly long life and its incalculable distance from her.

What had it seen in all its many years, way out there in space?

Jaina imagined that even stars had dreams, or maybe the entire universe itself was like a dream to them. After all, their perspective was so different from hers down on Earth.

As her eyelids began to close, lulled by the gentle hum of the moving car, she wondered just what it was like to look down from such a height....

When Jaina opened her eyes, she found that she was floating alone in the dark. No, not in the dark. A light shone in her face.

It took her eyes a moment to adjust.

She realized that she was looking up at the half-shadowed face of the moon, but it was so close! It filled nearly her whole field of vision.

She could almost reach out and touch it.

Jaina turned and saw below her the Earth in all its glory: blue and green, white swirling clouds forming pleasant shapes she recognized as birds, mice, flowers, and more.

Jaina just floated, breathlessly awed by the sight.

She had never realized how magnificent the world was, so vast in its infinite varieties and mysteries.

What a place to call home!

From here, she could even hear its song, a grand symphony formed by the smallest organism to the largest mountain in unison. Nothing could compare.

Another song called to her.

It was the Moon, a sweet note of admiration for the Earth that was its home as well. Jaina floated toward the moon and landed upon its surface.

It spoke to her in a voice that was both young and old, lilting and yet soothing. "Hello, little one. You travel far tonight. It pleases me that you can hear me sing to my greatest love."

Jaina beamed proudly. "Yes, I can! I have never heard the Moon like this before. Or the Earth. I am very happy to have gotten a chance to experience it. This is what it's like for you all the time?"

The Moon glowed happily. "The notes change depending on where I am, which is why I circle the whole world. I want to hear everything and everyone."

"Of course!" Jaina sprang lightly up, floating far above the surface of the moon. "I do, too. It is why I came out this far tonight. I really want to see what it's like outside of what I know."

"Then you will need to go very far tonight, little one! Let my gravity help you along, and remember to say goodnight when you come this way again." And the Moon exerted her gravity, propelling Jaina in a wide arc around her white surface.

Jaina laughed and cheered, feeling as though she was caught up in a sudden gust out in a place where no air existed. She waved farewell to the Moon as she sailed away.

A huge red planet greeted her with a bombastic song, like an entire orchestra of crashing cymbals and bellowing tubas.

Vast mountains and deep valleys scrawled across its surface gave the impression of a starkly rising and falling melody.

Craters pocked the surface, and in each one danced lights of peculiar color, always in some pattern.

Waves and snowflake-like formations, rippling circles, and stranger shapes appeared.
The dreams of Mars itself met with those of the people on Earth looking outward at the red planet, and the result was an aurora-like luminescence that blanketed the red planet. Thrilled, Jaina flew onward.

Far ahead, asteroids lay across her field of vision like dark flowers upon a starry black lawn.

Jaina swam freely through the open space to them, growing larger with each passing second.

There were small asteroids and medium-sized ones, and ones so huge they were like buildings floating in nothingness.

Some spun according to their own inertia, some floated motionlessly, and still, others turned this way and that.

Jaina landed upon one and found that she was not alone.

Little sprites danced merrily between pieces of asteroids, disappearing into one of the many holes in their porous surfaces only to emerge again with a cackle and a flash.

Jaina tried to follow them but they were too swift for her, ever urging her on with their laughter and frolicking.

Jaina leaped after one and it vanished in a puff, but she sailed into the tunnel into the asteroid.

Metals or gleaming crystals sparkled as she flew through a tunnel that rang with voices of fairies and capricious spirits of space and time.

Light-filled the tunnel like a sudden sun, but when she reached the other side, she found that she had only come back to the beginning.
The laughter of the fairies greeted her from within the tunnel.

Jaina laughed in turn. Their games were not malicious, just tricky.

"Okay, keep your secrets! I think I'm too big to fit, anyway!"

"Size is very relative here," said one of the spirits, appearing like a miniature ghostly star wreathed in cosmic dust.

In one moment, it was small as a baseball, and when Jaina blinked for that instant, the spirit seemed inconceivably vast as the Sun.

"In the dreams of the universe, 'big' or 'small' is meaningless. You are as important as the biggest asteroid, the smallest sun. The galaxy could not exist without you, and you could not exist without the galaxy!"

Jaina's eyes grew wide. "Oooh, I think I don't quite understand, but I want to!"

"Then journey further. All that is beckons you."

Jaina thanked the spirit and she drifted further still, past the asteroid belt.

As soon as she crossed that border, the music of the cosmos changed. It became loftier, more harmonic, and resonant in a way that reached into her deepest thoughts.

She closed her eyes and listened, content to be merely a part of the music of the spheres for a moment, an eternity.

When she opened her eyes again, she found that she had drifted near to a truly giant planet, a great swirling mass of browns and reds and cream colors, with a swirling eye roving this way and that.

Presently it turned to her, and she found that the world was speaking to her. Its voice was slow and sonorous, and it sounded a lot like the slow rush of an ocean wave.

"Welcome, traveler! What brings you out so far?"

Jaina grinned in pure pleasure. "Why, just seeing what the dreams above the clouds are like!"

Jupiter laughed a sound that rang across the entire solar system.

"Would you like to see what I see? Come into my eye and I will show you the things that even I dream about."

Excited beyond measure, Jaina flew toward the planet. "Yes, please! I want to see!"

As she dove into the great eye it became like a perfect rainstorm surrounding her, only the rain was made of soft light.

Winds swirled about her in a choir older than humanity itself, welcoming her, buoying her on their sweet serenade.

Then the swirling clouds broke and she saw with the planet's great eye. In an instant, her gaze was cast across the cosmos, beyond the planets of the solar system with their great icy rings and pale colors.

She saw to distant stars, which burned with a halo of colors, serpentine "sun dogs" coiling gracefully around them, and the myriad kaleidoscope shapes that appeared in their fiery surfaces.

Each one was a lens for the dreams of distant places, shining a light into the beautiful expanse of space.

Her gaze swung again and she saw to a vast maroon cloud unfolding. It looked like a giant bird unfurling its wings, speckled with stars like diamonds studding its feathers.

Its great fiery plume slowly expanded, the whole nebula growing like an eagle spreading its wings for the flight across the vastness of the cosmos.

Points of brilliant light appeared around it in great reddish-white flashes, and in each, one was born a new world of dreams.

The birdlike nebula opened its beak and uttered a cry of creation, and from its throat flowed the stuff of which worlds were made. Dust, gases, and matter flowed forth in a flood so titanic it would blanket a world, spiraling together, a burning ember at its heart. More joined the cosmic deluge and more still, and in the heart of it all, a star was born from the very dreams of the universe.

The bird-nebula spread its wings further and flew from one end of space to the other, trailing pure magic from its wings.

Comets and belts of stars and spinning rings floated outward from its wake, each going on to seek yet more places to manifest celestial phenomena.

Jaina in Jupiter's eye blinked and then it looked further still, watching a star in its final brilliant moments before it burst.

Impossibly bright, it is light-filled the firmament. Each ray carried the wishes of all who had looked upon a star and wished, each one forming from Dreamtime to scatter across the universe.

New paths were born for those who dreamed to reach the most far-flung of destinations, forged by the light of the dying star.

Even its magnificent ending created new life, for itself and for others, by filling the universe with newfound hope and inspiration.

Beyond the supernova lay a band of similar stars suspended in white mist. The whole of the Milky Way galaxy stretched out before her.

Its beating heart was a bright white center around which the entire Dreamtime world spiraled, all sharing the same space and time.

For here, there were no barriers between time and thought, spirit and space, dream and cosmic law.

Nebulae unfolded in silent compositions that told of the birth of entire worlds.
Stars emerged from the ether and grew into cosmic forges so hot that to strike upon them was to shape solar systems.

The majesty she witnessed expanding across the boundless universe was enough to forever touch Jaina's imagination.

Nothing she had ever dreamed prepared her for the scope and the power of the universe on this scale.

She swam in a vision of pure bliss borne upon the very spirit of the cosmos and felt its irresistible pull.

Cool blue stars glimmered in the clouds of reddish-white dust.

Planets swam through the great ocean of space, caught in the tides cast by the stars.

Comets soared through this like great travelers exploring worlds unknown.

The universal music reached from the very highest to the very smallest, leaving nothing untouched by its harmonies.

Light flowed across the known and unknown, hemmed by the dark of open space, a grand vision of timeless existence.

The most potent of possibilities collided with the least of impossibilities to bring forth the stuff of dreams and visions.

For each raindrop that fell upon an ocean, a star shone in the heavens and brought to light yet another facet of this incalculable grandness.

Jaina slept, completely enthralled by the visions of all that was and all that would one day exist, and how it sang from the very instruments of creation.

She felt her small part in that primordial music and she knew peace, oneness with the universe.

For only in a dream could someone know what it truly meant to be a part of it all, a wanderer in a place so incredible that it defied pure understanding, and yet never alone on the journey?

Every star in the universe shone its light upon her, and in turn, her every dream fed them. Every time she saw a star twinkle in the sky from that day forth, Jaina knew.

The stars were dreaming, too.

Travels

Through parallel dimensions
Travels in time and space
Seeking companionship without pretensions

Searching for a giver of much-needed advice
A keeper of secrets and dreams
Nothing else will suffice

Shall I find them running thru the park
Or perhaps getting lost on an adventure,
And ending up in an enchanted cave after dark

Through travels, I found a confidant and friend
A gentle, kindred soul
Who will travel unfettered through time, and space until the
end

Time?

Does it seem that you are stuck in the past?
You know the times are good, but they won't last.
Do you feel that you've lived in this time before?
And no matter what you, do the die has already been cast...

Does it feel that strangers are all the friends you used to know
And you left them in the future to come and watch this show
Of all the things you did and the person you used to be
Do you feel this too, or is it just me

Perhaps its already happened before we ever began
Maybe time is just a spiral and we're all just dancers
Going around and round
jumping back and forth looking for some answers

Floating through Space

I am weightless, a celestial flyer
I float passed planets, rising higher
I somersault and spin
This vast universe where does it begin?

Galaxies in the distance, I observe
A meteor on a collision course, I must swerve
Tumbling where there is not up or down
Stars, shooting all around

I soar and I swoop, taking in the worlds unknown
From one of them imitates and otherworldly tone
That planet there with the multi-colored rings
It has a voice, with an eerie melody, it sings

Floating through space, I am but a traveling soul
All of this wonder and beauty must extol
When at last, to my bed I must finally return
I close my eyes and sigh, and for the stars, I yearn

Shooting Star

I once took a ride upon a shooting star
I traveled so fast and so far,
I heard each and every with as it was made
And watched every dream as it was displayed

I once took a ride across the midnight sky
Soaring with glee, as I pretend to fly
Basking in the star's fiery glow
I watched with wonder at each village below

I once took a ride through my window and into my bed
I felt the droop of my eye and the nod of my head
Then away again, I rode to the land of dreams
To remember that magic is sometimes more than it seems

Chapter 10: Returning to Earth

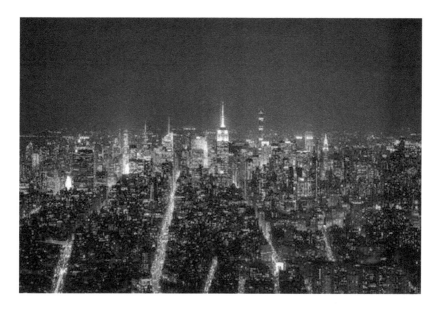

The kids were at last tucked in bed. The bags were unpacked and the clothes put away.

Jenny stood in the kitchen, holding a steaming hot mug of tea. She was exhausted from the long car ride and all the settling back in that they had to do, but she was glad to be home.

As much as she loved camping, and visiting the desert, the forest, and all the little wonderful mom-and-pop shops along the way, there was something about being home again that was a relief.

She had kicked her shoes off and now, with everyone else in the house asleep, it was her time to reflect.

After she had finished her tea, Jenny went upstairs and began to draw a hot bath.

She spilled lavender into the churning waters and at once, a soothing aroma filled the room.

Jenny had earned her time to relax, and as she stepped into the hot water, she knew that it was time to collect on it.

Laying back and resting her head back against the cool wall above the bathtub, Jenny took in several deep breaths of the lavender-scented steam.

Letting them slowly out, she looked up at the ceiling, noticing the faint brown water stains on the ceiling.

Jenny smiled and shook her head. Her husband was as bad with the splashing as the kids.

One of them was a spot with a short bar next to it, resembling the number "10."

She stared at it for a moment as her eyelids drooped with the weight of the day.

At last, she sighed and closed her eyes, and decided that she would let her mind wander a while.

The hot water cradled her body and soothed aching muscles. The steam refreshed her mind. Now she would let them help sweep her into a place of true relaxation.

Slipping into a light but blessed sleep, Jenny dreamed that she was another young woman in life both familiar and different, another time, another place, dreaming the same dreams....

* * *

Jaina lay beneath an open window with a fan blowing softly upon her. Sounds drifted in through the apartment window.

Outside, the city was alive despite the late hour. A honking horn in the distance. A truck rumbling past. A lone cat's exploratory meow. The steady drip of moisture from a gutter pipe. The wind in the leaves outside, and rushing through the alleyways with a soft whisper. All were part of the music of the city.

Jaina saw them more clearly now, deep within a peaceful sleep in her bed.

A cat walked proudly in one of the alleyways.

This was his home, and he knew every corner like it was another whisker on his face.

Every garbage can, every fence, every open window with its tempting treats.
For the cat could see the dreams of the sleepers in his domain, and he often flitted in and out of their dreams as well.

Cats knew the paths between the hidden and unhidden better than most.

Their eyes could see that which remained just out of sight in the yellow glare of the streetlights, in the deep shadows that lay between alleys and beneath doorsteps.

The cat wandered because it could feel the tug of those invisible threads and like a kitten chasing a ball of yarn he wanted to bat at them, chase them, and even pounce upon the possibilities with the vigor only the young knew.

What better a place to call home than the places between worlds when one had the grace of a cat?

The cat was not alone. A crow perched atop a power line watching him with bemused curiosity. She knew the same hidden realms he did, for her eyes saw them.

Few could find their way between the worlds like crows, who were born with a gift for it.

When she flew, the wind that blew beneath her wings traveled in and out of the dreams of the city, and so did the crow herself.

She saw the city as it saw itself, its truest reflection.

Beyond the veils where weary but wakeful people walked, the city came to life in a way that only those who slept deeply could possibly understand.

The crow sometimes guided others to that world, but just as often the city itself did. She flew from her perch and from her bird's eye view, she lives in motion.

Spirits in the wind loved to cavort above the rooftops and down in the alleys, where they could stir up a commotion and playfully tease the cats, the rats, the crawling critters, and those who slept with their windows open.

Jaina heard them and stirred in her sleep, but she saw with dreaming eyes their carefree antics, just as the crow did.

The dreams of a city were as myriad as its own population.

Streets of endless beauty, the roads shining as though studded with diamonds, each streetlight like a torch in a misty night.

Doorways opened into a warm glow were rooms that had seen generations passed still echoed with laughter and mirth.

Entire buildings resonated with the hopes and passions of those who dwelt within, and those dreams like water-soaked down to the roots, and so the city bloomed.

While those insides slumbered, the hidden things came out to enjoy the world they had created.

Sprites and spirits of the urban landscape emerged to dance in the trees, or frolic along the sidewalks, and bound into every open window.

Their celebrations touched the whole city and imbued it with a sense of hope for tomorrow.

Those who dreamed filled blank windows with their light, or sent a refreshing gust down the streets and the city welcomed them all. Its life and legacy were born of those very dreams.

Rats in the alleyway cried an energetic farewell as the cat approached them.
 They plunged into the cracks that opened up into great tunnels beneath the world the people knew.

The labyrinth became an intricate maze where countless furry rodents sang happily.

They sang of food, freedom, and family. Theirs was an entire kingdom to themselves and often took them through the beautiful and strange worlds of dreaming people.

A tunnel may open onto a forest grove or a canyon vista, might echo with the crash of ocean surf, or lead to a banquet where the finest foods had been laid out for them.

One door could lead to the stars themselves, or emerge from a knot in a tree looking down upon a field full of colorful flowers.

Into this maze of possibilities, they happily wove, finding therein glimpses at many things they had never known.

Capricious fairies danced merrily upon the outside window ledges. They plucked images from the dreams of those just inside and gently cast them through the windows, where they would form star fields and baseball fields and wheat fields.

The sleepers would be transported into the worlds their innermost desires sought to explore.

A smile stole across their lips as a sensation more real than imagined caressed their outstretched hands or whispered faint words of becoming.

Those lucky sleepers awoke the next day to find that their dreams had come true in some way, big or small, and still the city grew.

A couple walked down the street arm in arm, and their soft voices mingled together like the background song of an old restaurant. They could have been anyone, or no one at all, a reflection of the lives built in the city over the decades.

Those who heard them knew that they were not alone, no matter how late the hour, for someone else lived and dreamed in the city.

Before them, the sidewalk was a well-illumined path into the heart of the city, where neon signs flashed to welcome people into warmly lit diners and a bell rang somewhere every time a door opened.

The clatter of a cup and saucer met with the swish of a coat or the creak of a padded bench.

The car that cruised the streets may have had no driver, nor needed one. For those whose dreams took them to the road, it was a carriage.

Maybe it was an early morning vacation road trip, laden with excitement at the possibilities ahead.

Perhaps a return from a late-night movie outing, or a lover's home, aglow with the experience of the night.

Perhaps a child slept in the backseat, lulled into a peaceful sleep by the gentle motion of the car.

The city welcomed them all, who had built it brick by brick, dream by dream, since its inception.

Stacks of newspapers were tossed into kiosks and trunks, crinkling as their handlers bound them in rubber bands.

Each carried tales from across the city and much further, each bound for different destination, but always to end up in someone's hands. In the early hours, where steam and fog drifted through the streets, the paper deliverers whistled their work songs and prepared for their daily routes.

These early hours were the most peaceful; while most of the city slept, they were awake and full of energy. They prepared to bring the day's news to those who were united by the threads of shared stories.

A dog whined happily as his owner returned from a late shift. The dog stood with its paws up on the windowsill, watching his best friend walk to the door, and greeted him with many happy tail wags.

For the dog, the dream only started when his owner had returned, and now could return to more pleasant things like biscuits, open-window car rides, and days spent running through the park.

But he would sleep by his owner's bed tonight and guard his dreams, for they often ran together through the worlds beyond sleep. There neither of them would tire, and treats would rain aplenty for all. For the dog and his owner alike, the city was home, and they loved it.

Jaina heard this music, the most discordant of all, and yet not less beautiful.
For the many facets, some of the odd or out of place, that made up the sleeping city fit together all the better for their seeming clashes.

The car that rattled by with a squeaky belt was as calming as the sound of doves outside the window in its own way.

It told of another series of stories.

How did the car come to be that way?

Who drove it now and who before that?

Where must it be going?

Beyond all these questions, the car bore the dreams of the one who drove it.

For that person, too, had dreams of their own, whether leaving home or returning to it, seeking a new possibility or meeting an old one.

One simple trip to the store meant questions and answers in equal measure to those who heard the sputtering song of a beat-up old car.

In the great city parks, statues stood silent in the night, save to those who slept and could hear their songs. Each resonated with its own music, standing like beacons to those who walked the dreaming paths.

Therefore, visitors did, welcomed by the statues whose unflinching smiles and enduring tunes anchored travelers. Built to help guide the imaginations of all who came to them, the statues beyond the wall of sleep were anything but rigid.

They bore hopes upon their shoulders, they fostered inspiration, and they carried the wishes of all who had cast pennies into their fountains, or looked up at them and marveled.

Pathways wove throughout the park, in the magical night like sheet music littered with notes.

The right footsteps would play the traveler upon a musical path that could guide her right into the pulse of the city itself. Pigeons cooed in the branches above, creating a lilting but sweet symphony that blended well with the extended notes played along the paths.

Here, the city welcomed the dreams of the green growing things into its midst, encompassing those within and those without.

Following these paths led Jaina to an ornate public fountain at the center of the park.

Water plumed upward and cascaded down, catching rainbows in the beams of the streetlights.

The gurgle of the water in the basin spoke excitedly of every single wish ever made upon it, and the copper and silver coins shining within each carried a piece of a life's story.

For the thousands of coins cast with a wish into the fountain painted a picture, the mosaic of lives that formed the city itself.

No one person could fill such a place alone, but the city thrived on their dreams *en masse*.

Each one brick or a block of foundation, a pane of glass in a window like an eye into the city's life.

Each footstep, each word another part of the urban orchestra.

All of the places Jaina had visited in her sleep were unique, but the city perhaps the most unique of all.

For it was not born of any one thing, nor did it display a single kind of view, image, fantasy.

It was a composite of all of these things, and all the competing notes simply subsumed into the city's overall tune.

In it, there were people whose dreams took them to the stars and beyond, into the furthest depths of space.

Others ventured nightly through the wilds of the deserts, where rain was a miracle and the warmth of the day evaporated into a chilly but fascinating night.

Some might wander over the tundra, over snow and ice, where lights in the sky were less bright than the very land itself, and living things thrived in the snowy plains.

Birds on the wing and dolphins in the salty waves enjoyed the same company, whether the dreamer lay upon a white sand shore or safely tucked away in bed in a third-floor apartment.

Autumn came to the city, as well, golden and fair, and so did the white winters lit by the warm glow of lights within.

Spring saw growth in the city's people. New businesses flourished. New lives were born. New bonds forged. New dreams realized.

When summers bloomed, the city flushed with heat and commotion, never sleeping even in the latest of hours.
For Jaina, life in the city contained pieces of everything she had ever known. Every dream she had ever experienced found its way here.

She had grown through those dreams into a young woman capable of standing on her own, but most importantly, she had never forgotten where they came from.

They were a part of her, each an important part of the music that made her the person that she had become—and helped compose the person she would be in the future.

Here, she never felt alone. Whether it was hers or someone else's, she always had the company of a dream to guide her through restful sleep.

The city never slept, but it was always dreaming.

Bedtime Routine

When the night has fallen and is ready to settle
I get out the tea and heat the kettle
A hot bubble bath to soak away the aches and pains

And then, jammie clad, tea in my hand, I head for my chair
I light a candle lavender and sandalwood scents fill the air
All the cozier this in on a night when it rains

I wrap a handmade quilt around tight
Picking up my book, I let my imagination take flight
My mind ventures through worlds I have never visited before

At last, sleepy-eyed, I nestle into my bed to sleep
To the world of dreams, now I creep
Continuing the adventures, in the worlds, my mind wishes to
explore.

My City

At night I walk down the city street
The neon glow lights the path before me
This is my city, at night, alive.

The vibrancy of the night is the city's heartbeat
And everywhere I look is something new to see
In my city, this is where I thrive

Skyscrapers kiss the night skyline
Lights twinkling from every storefront window
Music wafting on the wind, from some unseen merrymakers

This is home, this city, it is mine
In my veins, I feel its ebb and flow
I wouldn't trade my city for a thousand country acres

Cityscape

One sleepless night, I looked out my window
On the twenty-fourth floor
I admired the cityscape below

High rise buildings lit from within
Reaching to the night heavens
At their feet, a lonely musician playing his violin

A young couple walks close, arms entwined
A first date, or a well-established love?
Or possibly a relationship of another kind?

A stray cat scurries across their path
Chasing a mouse, or some other creature
That has invoked his wrath.

Closing the curtain, I return to my bed
I think, that now I may sleep
With the rhythm of the cityscape playing in my head

My Cat

My cat spends his day lying in the sun
And chasing dust motes for fun
He purrs for attention
And meows to show his condescension

He falls asleep soundly in my lap
Never mind if I have things to do, he needs a nap
But when he wants to play
He is a fierce predator, and nothing stands in his way

Bedtime finds him snoozing there on my bed
No, not at the foot, up at the head
Dreaming his feline dreams
All of the worlds is his, or so it seems

CPSIA information can be obtained
at www.ICGtesting.com
Printed in the USA
LVHW011108301020
670159LV00013B/509